NAPOLI

MW00824567

Specs Appeal

Extravagant 1950s and 1960s Eyewear

PHOTOGRAPHY AND DESIGN BY LESLIE PIÑA
TEXT BY DONALD-BRIAN JOHNSON

Anita —
Thank you for keeping
us looking good all of
these years!
Sincerely,
Laurie Haslund

PROJECT COORDINATOR: LAURIE HASLUND
RESEARCH ASSOCIATES: BARBARA WARD ENDTER,
ELLEN FOSTER, & JOSE VEGA
ADDITIONAL PHOTOGRAPHY: ELIOT CROWLEY
PHOTOGRAPHY ASSOCIATE: RAMÓN PIÑA

Schiffer Publishing Ltd ®

4880 Lower Valley Road, Atglen, PA 19310 USA

DEDICATION

For Chuck and Cathleen Johnson, Paul, Mary, and Sarah.

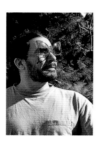

Layout by Bonnie M. Hensley
Type set in Korinna BT

ISBN: 0-7643-1403-3
Printed in China
1 2 3 4

Published by Schiffer Publishing Ltd.
4880 Lower Valley Road
Atglen, PA 19310
Phone: (610) 593-1777; Fax: (610) 593-2002
E-mail: Schifferbk@aol.com
Please visit our web site catalog at **www.schifferbooks.com**
We are always looking for people to write books on new and related subjects. If you have an idea for a book please contact us at the above address.

This book may be purchased from the publisher.
Include $3.95 for shipping.
Please try your bookstore first.
You may write for a free catalog.

In Europe, Schiffer books are distributed by
Bushwood Books
6 Marksbury Ave.
Kew Gardens
Surrey TW9 4JF England
Phone: 44 (0) 20 8392-8585; Fax: 44 (0) 20 8392-9876
E-mail: Bushwd@aol.com
Free postage in the U.K., Europe; air mail at cost.

CONTENTS

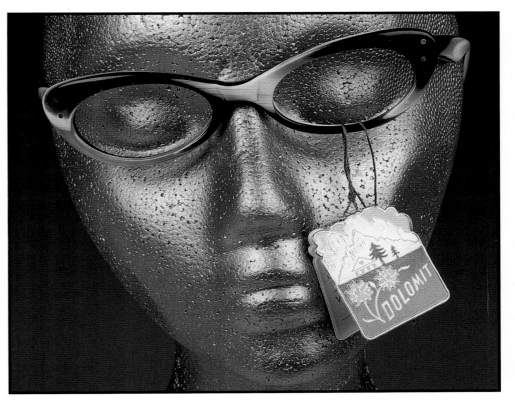

ACKNOWLEDGMENTS

Our sincere appreciation to Laurie Haslund, Coast to Coast Collections, for suggesting and promoting the development of this project. Her knowledge of fashion eyewear and wealth of collector contacts have proven invaluable. Our gratitude, as well, to the many eyewear manufacturers and designers of the 1950s and 1960s, whose imaginative creations defined "specs appeal."

Thanks also to the following, who have contributed their collections, expertise, encouragement—or a blend of all three—to *Specs Appeal*: Ken Able; Marilyn Cohen, The Marilyn Cohen Collection; Eliot Crowley Photography; Barbara Ward Endter; Dale Endter; Alana Fornoni, Alana: Antique & Estate Jewelry; Ellen Foster, Vanity Lady; Tim Holthaus & Jim Petzold, Ceramic Arts Studio Collectors Association; Charles M. Johnson, Sr., and Patricia P. Johnson; Hank Kuhlmann; Vicki Lynn; Andrea Macaione; Office Depot Omaha; Ramón Piña; Gary Piper; Jose Vega, and, of course, Peter Schiffer, Douglas Congdon-Martin, Bonnie M. Hensley, and the staff at Schiffer Publishing. Without each of you, *Specs Appeal* would have been less spec-tacular!

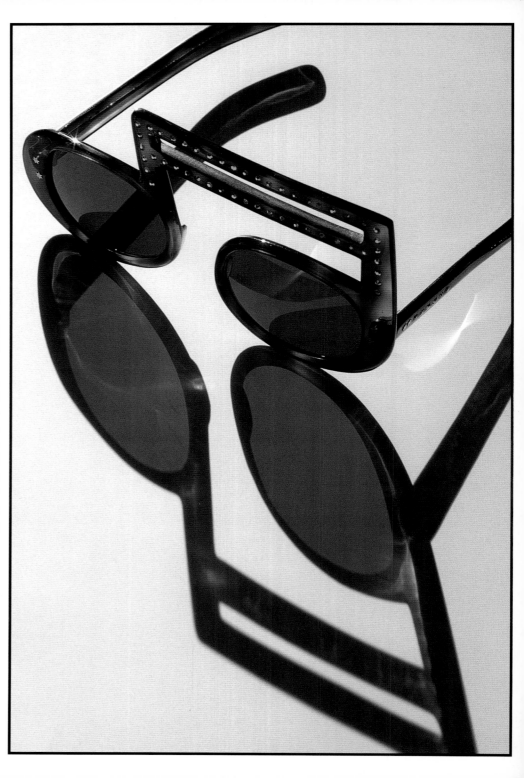

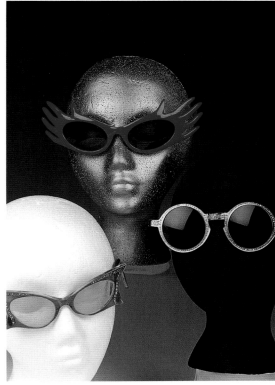

Chapter 1:
"ONE PAIR IS NOT ENOUGH"

Eyewear: From Functional To Fashionable

Men seldom make passes at girls who wear glasses.
—Dorothy Parker

Ms. Parker's mid-twentieth century quote just put into words what many had been thinking for years. "Glasses" and "glamorous" were terms never used in tandem. Girls without glasses were wives and sweethearts. Girls with glasses were spinsters and maiden aunts. Girls without glasses hit the dance floors. Girls with glasses hit the books. Ruby Keeler, in glasses, was a secretary. Ruby Keeler, once that wise producer in *Footlight Parade* whipped off her glasses and revealed Ruby's pretty face, was the toast of Broadway. Wonder Woman's secret identity wore glasses. Wonder Woman didn't.

In short, glasses, until mid-century, were regarded as a necessary evil—a medical necessity—a means of avoiding the annoyance of bumping into things or whispering sweet nothings to total strangers. People wore glasses because they had to. Those afflicted gave no more thought to the concept of "fashionable" glasses than they did to the concept of fashionable dentures. Glasses were what they were—and what they were was not very appealing.

It wasn't always so. In the 1700s, the height of fashionable dress always included some form of often impractical eyewear—from "scissors glasses" to luridly colored lenses to the "Quizzer," an affectation on the order of a magnifying glass. However, as the Industrial Revolution of the mid-1800s made glasses affordable for the mass market, the emphasis shifted from style to serviceability. The choice of a frame was generally left to the optician, much as the choice of a prescribed medicine was left to the family doctor.

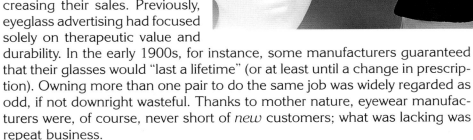

In the mid-1900s, "fashionable" once more took precedence over "functional." The reason was simple: eyewear manufacturers realized that increasing their potential market meant increasing their sales. Previously, eyeglass advertising had focused solely on therapeutic value and durability. In the early 1900s, for instance, some manufacturers guaranteed that their glasses would "last a lifetime" (or at least until a change in prescription). Owning more than one pair to do the same job was widely regarded as odd, if not downright wasteful. Thanks to mother nature, eyewear manufacturers were, of course, never short of *new* customers; what was lacking was repeat business.

Bringing them back for more meant that eyeglass design had to reflect, complement, and ultimately embrace the taste of the times. In 1930, the industry took its first steps toward fashion respectability, as models donned glasses for a major fashion show at New York's Waldorf-Astoria. Then, in 1939, Altina Sanders premiered her "Harlequin" frame. Regarded as the first real fashion frame design, the "Harlequin" won an America Design Award for its creator and was a precursor of the upswept cat-eye frames so prevalent in the 1950s.

With the intervention of World War II, fashion was placed on a back burner, as development efforts were directed to the war effort. Wartime inventiveness, however, paid off when peacetime arrived. Thanks to war-related research, cellulose acetate emerged as a stable (and affordable) frame option.

Since the late 1800s, various thermoplastic materials which would successfully hold a desired shape had been used as an alternative to all-wire glasses. (The first such product was DuPont's "Zylonite," and "Zyl" is still used by the eyewear industry today, as an all-purpose term for plastic.) Nitrate, introduced in the 1920s, had allowed for the production of more colorful frames—but nitrate was expensive, hard to work with, and worst of all, flammable. Cellulose acetate was a welcome, workable alternative, and in 1948 Bay State Optical introduced the first molded frame. Eyewear, as fashion, was finally on the move!

While most remember the 1950s for cat-eye overkill and rhinestone excess, the decade's most significant development for everyday eyeglass wear was really the browbar, or "combination frame;" it colorfully combined plastic tops with metal rims. Also zooming into view in the '50s was the first "designer line" of frames, courtesy of Schiaparelli. Since then, designers from Cassini to Pucci have created signature eyewear, but Schiaparelli was there first, in a 1955 collaboration with American Optical.

Soon, repeat business was booming, thanks to advertising campaigns by such manufacturers as Bausch & Lomb. B & L bombarded optical offices with promos firmly declaring "One Pair of Glasses is Not Enough." To drive home the point, the company in 1953 crowned its first "Miss Specs Appeal;" the honor was awarded to "America's prettiest model who wears glasses." Miss Specs and her successors (the more demurely titled "Miss Beauty in Glasses") proudly told anyone who would listen that the secret to "specs appeal" was wearing fashionable glasses—and plenty of them. As a guest on Steve Allen's TV show, 1954's winner, Libby Booth, authoritatively stated, "modern frames for various occasions are as much a part of fashion today as shoes, hats, or jewelry." Among her personal collection, Libby counted Hi-Lites, Balrims, Cordelles, and Ray-Bans—all, of course, by B & L. Glasses, as fashion, had arrived.

Throughout the 1950s and '60s, the notion of glasses as a choice—something that, while practical, could still enhance attractiveness—took hold.

In 1961, the Fashion Eyewear Group of America (FEGA) was established. By 1962, an entire section of *Vogue* focused on fashionable eyewear. Over the years, glasses became seen as an outward manifestation of the inner personality, with celebrities as diverse as Jacqueline Onassis, Elton John, and Dame Edna Everage readily identifiable by a "look" that prominently featured distinctive eyewear. Even those who didn't need glasses snapped them up, with most styles available in both prescription and "plano."

Today, retro tastes influence new styles, as evidenced by the Alain Mikli "Barbie Eyewear" line of 1999: just like Barbie wore, in shades of hot pink, with the addition of Barbie-Doll legs as temples! Additionally, many eyewear styles of the twentieth century have direct counterparts in the twenty-first: metal ovals of the 1920s...geometrics and rounds from the '30s...1940s tortoise-shells...'50s bejeweled plastics...'60s designer lines...oversized, overcolored 1970s frames...and 1980s tailored "yuppie" styles, "total fashion looks," and sport-specific "performance" sunwear. All of these are echoed in the vintage eyewear recreations and adaptations which began in the 1990s and have continued into the new millennium.

For eyewear collectors, the retro revival has been an ideal opportunity to resuscitate the past, making it work for today. Frames of previous eras are eagerly sought out, then taken to an optician, and either reborn as sun glasses or fitted with the wearer's own prescription for everyday use. Some collectors take pride in owning a pair of glasses for every occasion—from oversize "butterfly" frames for the splashiest of evenings out to sun glasses with their own working awnings (giving new meaning to the term "shades").

For 1950s eyewear manufacturers, "one pair is not enough" was a sales booster. For today's collectors, it's become a rule to live by. Our own "blast from the past" begins now. Put on your specs and page through *Specs Appeal*, revisiting those whimsical designs of bygone days. Chances are good you'll find something that will catch your eye. And remember: "one pair of glasses is not enough!"

Opposite page: "Specs appeal:" in the 1950s, it captured the nation's fancy. As this American Optical Company ad notes, eyeglasses were at last regarded as "smart fashion accessories...designed by stylists as carefully as a Paris original to flatter your eyes—compliment your coloring—really *do* something for you." Poor granny. Her glasses only helped her see better!

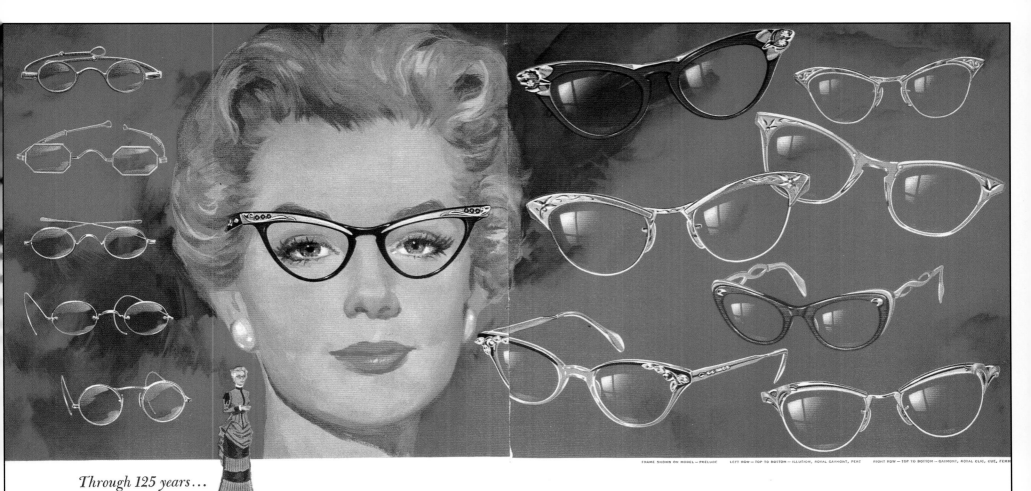

FRAME SHOWN ON MODEL — PRELUDE   LEFT ROW — TOP TO BOTTOM — ILLUSION, ROYAL GAYMONT, PERT   RIGHT ROW — TOP TO BOTTOM — GAYMONT, ROYAL CLIC, CUE, FEMM

Through 125 years...

Grandma's "Specs" Have Become *Today's Fashion Showpieces*

When American Optical first started making silver-framed glasses in 1833, folks didn't think about how the *frames* looked. They were just downright glad to see better.

But how things have changed. Today, glasses not only help you see better, but American Optical frames are smart fashion accessories . . . designed by stylists as carefully as a Paris original. Frames are scientifically sound and glow with fashion's warmest colors . . .

gleam with sparkling trim. Best of all, American Optical frames flatter your eyes . . . compliment your coloring . . . really *do* something for you.

You can obtain these new American Optical Showpieces anywhere in America through the Eye Care Professions.

RED DOT An AO exclusive.

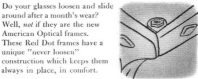

Do your glasses loosen and slide around after a month's wear? Well, *not* if they are the new American Optical frames. These Red Dot frames have a unique "never loosen" construction which keeps them always in place, in comfort.

BETTER VISION FOR BETTER LIVING

American Optical
COMPANY
SOUTHBRIDGE, MASSACHUSETTS

©1958 AMERICAN OPTICAL COMPANY

7

Eyeing the Past

While *Specs Appeal* focuses on the popular, rather than the historical, aspects of eyewear, here's a brief glimpse back at several outstanding optical occurrences:

350 B.C.: Aristotle complains about his eyes.

1268 or **1287** or **Sometime Prior:** depending on which reference you go by, eyewear first became known through the writings of Roger Bacon in 1268—or by drawings dating from northern Italy in 1287—or in China at some prior time unknown, since medieval illustrations exist of Chinese people in glasses. In any event, it was too late for Aristotle.

Mid-1300s: Convex lenses, made of beryl or quartz, come into use and solve a host of vision problems. (But unless you're nobility or clergy, they're not for you.)

1352: Cardinal Hugh of Provence (see? clergy) bravely lets Tommaso da Modena paint him with his glasses on. A first.

1666: Home remedies, courtesy of Robert Turner: "for squint, the blood of a turtle or head of a bat, powdered, of course. For weak sight, the eyes of a cow hung around the neck."

1700s: That's why they call them "temples": to keep glasses on the head, sidebars are added. And they reach as far as the temples.

1784: Ben Franklin invents bifocals, cleverly combining glass halves of different strengths, making one pair of glasses do the work of two.

1853: Mr. Bausch meets Mr. Lomb. For $60 each, the fellas share half interest in a tray of optical blanks and frames. They soon own more.

1850s: A revolutionary development: glazed lenses, a product of the Industrial Revolution, make eyeglasses available to a mass market.

1868: "Here's your prescription, sir." The first-ever doctor-given Rx for spectacles is presented to William Y. McAllister by Dr. Dyer (along with his bill).

1880s: Temples make it the rest of the way, adding earpieces.

1909: The first all-artificial plastic is introduced, meaning eyeglass frames will finally stay in adjustment. Better yet, it comes in lots of colors!

1929: A group with a vision: the Better Vision Institute (BVI) is formed.

1930: Fresh-faced models cover those fresh faces with eyeglasses, in a first-ever fashion show featuring eyewear.

1939: Altina Sanders creates the "Harlequin." A nation of grateful cat-eye lovers says "meow."

1947: *Business Week* takes note of the "teen-age rebellion against the solemn, round, owl-eyed type of horn-rims." Fortunately, the introduction of cellulose acetate means molded cat-eye frames will soon be giving all teens "paws" to reflect.

1953: "Miss Specs Appeal" receives her crown (and a nice selection of free frames), boldly declaiming "one pair of glasses is not enough." Time proves her right.

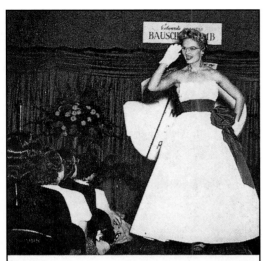

Above: She earned her keep! When Bausch & Lomb selected Nancy Ann Miller as the first "Miss Specs Appeal" in 1953, one prize was a trip to New York City.. While there, Nancy Ann appeared on TV, was interviewed on radio, and of course headlined a Bausch & Lomb fashion show, modeling the new "rhinestone-studded Cordelle glasses for evening."

Top center: Hailed as "America's prettiest model who wears glasses," Nancy Ann also received $300 in defense bonds, and a nice assortment of B & L frames.

Bottom center: After her hectic day, Miss Specs enjoyed a night on the town with escort Robert Q. Lewis (of radio fame). Thanks to Bausch & Lomb, both had no problem reading the menu!

Top right: Back to the beginning: long before Miss Specs was a twinkle in anyone's eye, less glamorous means promoted eyewear. These somewhat forbidding spectacle signs were available to opticians of the 1890s, from Spencer Optical. To complement the "handsome eye painted on each panel," buyers could add their name "neatly lettered in red," for just $1 extra.

Bottom right: Once lured inside, optical customers could have their vision checked with "Spencer's Opthalmoscopic Test Lenses," guaranteed to "detect all visual defects" including "near sight, far sight, old sight and poor sight."

Vol. 13 · No. 5   NOVEMBER-DECEMBER 1953

Balco News

FOR THE MEN AND WOMEN OF BAUSCH & LOMB OPTICAL COMPANY

U. S. CONTEST WINNER — "MISS SPECS APPEAL OF 1953"

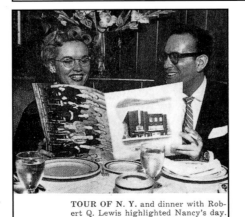

TOUR OF N. Y. and dinner with Robert Q. Lewis highlighted Nancy's day.

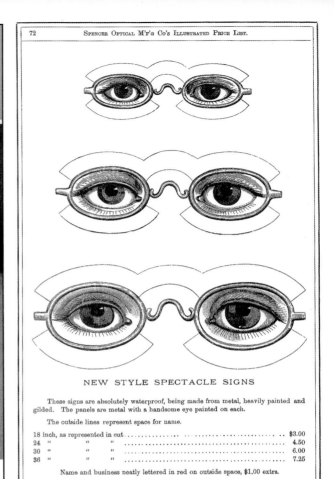

72   SPENCER OPTICAL M'F'G CO's ILLUSTRATED PRICE LIST.

NEW STYLE SPECTACLE SIGNS

These signs are absolutely waterproof, being made from metal, heavily painted and gilded. The panels are metal with a handsome eye painted on each.

The outside lines represent space for name.

18 inch, as represented in cut		$3.00
24 " " "		4.50
30 " " "		6.00
36 " " "		7.25

Name and business neatly lettered in red on outside space, $1.00 extra.

Spencer's Opthalmoscopic Test Lenses.

WILL DETECT ALL VISUAL DEFECTS.

A scientific and practical instrument, for detecting all optical defects of the eye and determining the lenses needed for their correction.

Use this instrument in adjusting Spectacles and Eye-Glasses in all cases of

MYOPIA, or Near Sight, — **HYPEROPIA,** or Far Sight, — **PRESBYOPIA,** or Old Sight, and **ASTIGMATISM,** or Poor Sight.

Caused by oval eyes which causes some figures on a clock dial, at fifteen feet, to look darker than others.

This instrument has the following advantages:

I. It is very ornamental and more attractive than any other instrument.

II. It measures all optical defects of the eye more rapidly and accurately than any other instrument.

III. It is the only instrument where the error due to the distance of the lenses from the eye is properly compensated for.

IV. It is the only instrument which, in addition to measuring the optical defect of the eye, measures instantly and in a satisfactory manner the exact distance between the pupils, and determines any weakness in the muscles which move the eyes.

V. The axis of the concave and convex cylindrical lenses are presented to the eye in the position they are most frequently required, 180 and 90 degrees respectively.

VI. It is much cheaper than any other instrument of the kind.

Price reduced to.................. $25.00

9

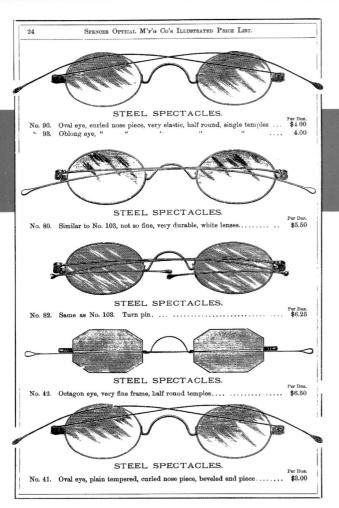

In less fashion-conscious times, eyeglass prices were unbelievably low. Spencer's least expensive steel spectacles sold wholesale at just $3—per dozen!

Top center: Other manufacturers of the time also offered optical bargains, tempting buyers with such phrases as "reduced price list" and "proportionately low prices." Budget-minded advertisers in this 1892 notice from *The Optical Journal* include L. Manasse Co., Otto Young, and Pacific Optical.

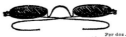
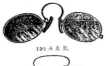
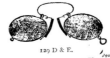
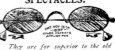
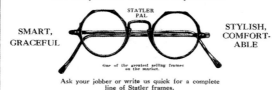 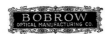
The WESTERN
OPTICAL WORLD

VOLUME IV   NUMBER X

April 1918

Gordon Grant

WILL YOU supply EYES for the NAVY?

An eye for an eye? Opticians of the World War I era received a patriotic jolt with this grim appeal for support. It appeared on the cover of the *The Western Optical World* in April, 1918.

By the 1920s, "inexpensive" and "practical" were no longer the most effective selling points for eyewear. New buzz words included "smart—graceful—stylish—comfortable." Bobrow's "Statler Pal," advertised in the September 26, 1929 issue of *The Optometric Weekly* was all of these and more, making it "one of the greatest selling frames on the market."

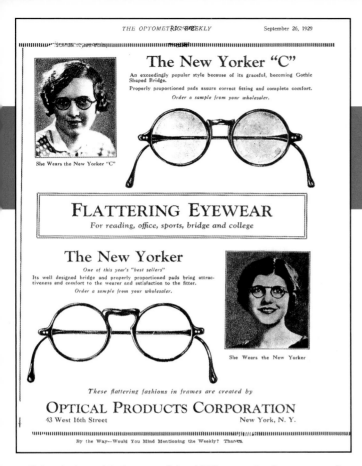

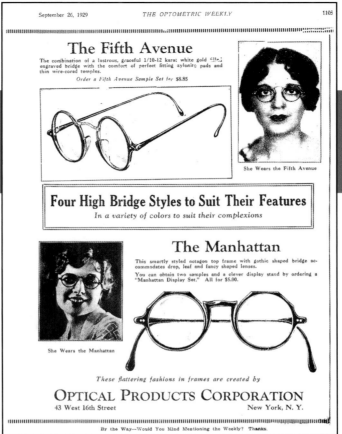

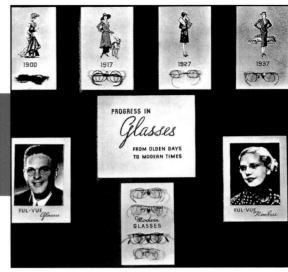

"From olden days to modern times:" in 1940, an American Optical Company display offered this glimpse of the 20th century's eyewear-progress-to-date. The 1950s were straight ahead...and eye-popping changes were in store!

Other fashionable frames of the 1920s promised a cosmopolitan touch. The names—"The New Yorker," "The Fifth Avenue," and "The Manhattan"—hinted at smart, big-city style. These Optical Products Corporation designs appeared in *The Optometric Weekly*, September 26, 1929.

11

50s Eyewear:
A Bird's-Eye View From B & L

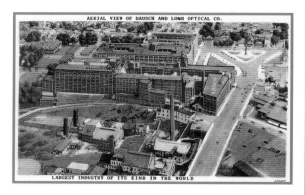

Top & bottom left: As the '50s dawned, one of the eyewear industry's largest manufacturers celebrated its 100th anniversary. Bausch & Lomb, the Rochester, New York-based giant, marked the occasion with a special centennial booklet. Photos and captions in this section, drawn from B & L's *A New Century*, offer a glimpse of eyewear manufacture and eye care as it existed in the early 1950s.

Top right: "Here is the prescription surfacing department in a modern ophthalmic laboratory. Many other departments and operations are necessary in the competent execution of the patient's prescription."

Bottom center: "Your visual correction is determined by an examination using several precise ophthalmic instruments designed by B & L engineers and produced by B & L craftsmen."

Bottom right: "For a hundred years, spectacle lenses have comprised one of the most important lines of Bausch & Lomb products. Every lens prescribed is one of several dozen types, in one of several hundred 'powers.'"

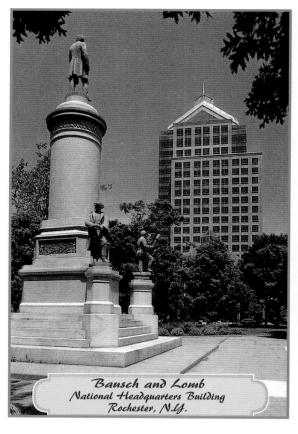

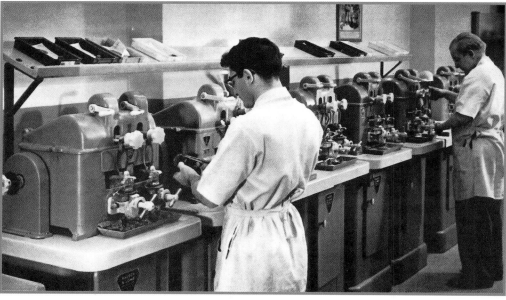

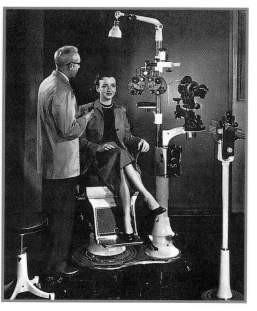

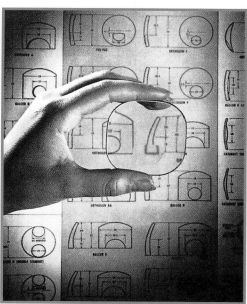

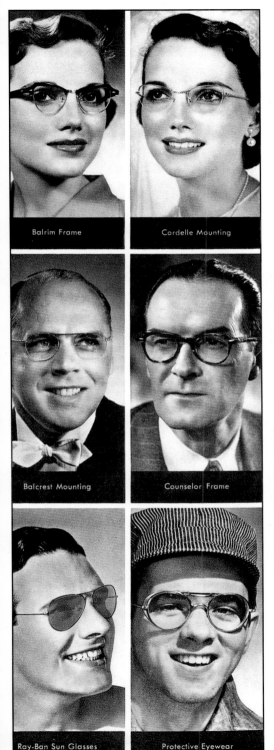

Balrim Frame

Cordelle Mounting

Balcrest Mounting

Counselor Frame

Ray-Ban Sun Glasses

Protective Eyewear

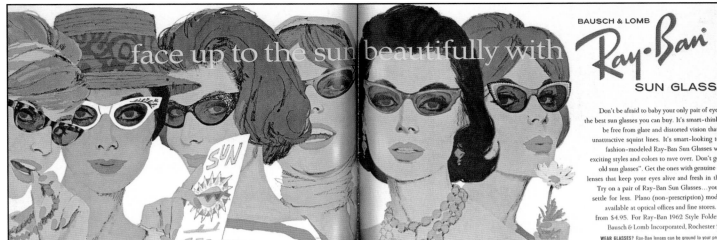

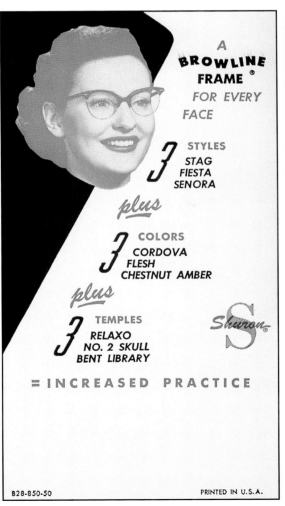

A
BROWLINE
FRAME ©
FOR EVERY
FACE

3 STYLES
STAG
FIESTA
SENORA

plus

3 COLORS
CORDOVA
FLESH
CHESTNUT AMBER

plus

Shuron®

3 TEMPLES
RELAXO
NO. 2 SKULL
BENT LIBRARY

= INCREASED PRACTICE

B28-850-50   PRINTED IN U.S.A.

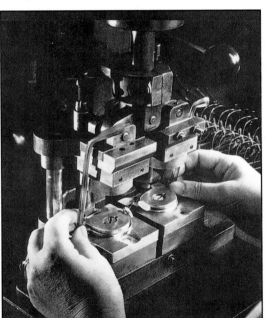

Top left: "Today, a lifetime of keen non-tiring vision is possible. In the mirror of the past, we see the image of the future. To that future—that eyes may see better—we dedicate our Centennial." A Bausch & Lomb hundredth anniversary frame sampler, 1953.

Bottom center: Forging forward into the '50s, B & L and its competitors—from American Optical to Willson—made "specs appeal" a priority. No more staid steel spectacles or prim "New Yorkers." Now, consumers browsed through such zestily titled selections as these by Shuron: "Stag," "Fiesta," and "Señora." The exotic shades offered ranged from "cordova" to "chestnut amber." The future beckoned...

Right: ...and so did the market for sun glasses. Whether the choice was prescription or "plano," consumers were advised "don't be afraid to baby your only pair of eyes." A major player in mid-century eyewear, sun glasses were available, according to Ray-Ban, in "frame styles so flattering they're almost wicked!" Now *that's* "specs appeal!"

Bottom right: "The manufacture of spectacle frames calls for metals of proper stamina and resiliency, and production methods of extreme precision. The spectacle frame or rimless mounting to hold the lenses correctly before your eyes—and to be well-styled and pleasing in appearance—may be of gold-filled metal or plastic or a combination of both."

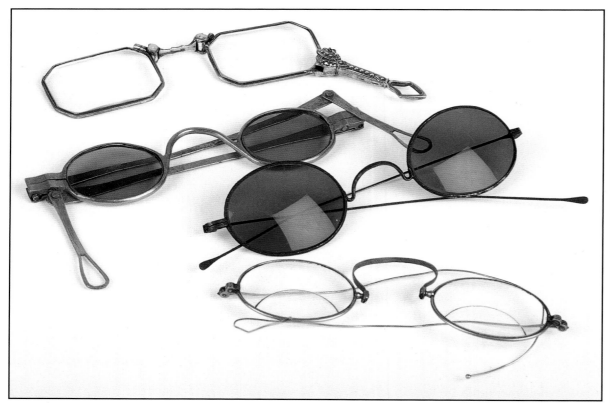

Spectacles through the centuries: a whirlwind tour of eyeglass stylings, past to present!

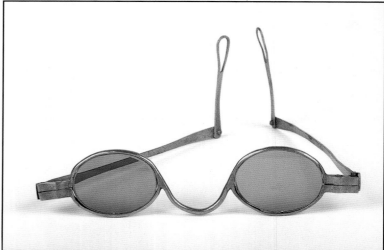

Top right: Circa 1727: wig glasses. Oval rings at the ends of the temples kept glasses in place under each profusely powdered head, while colored lenses had the wearer "seeing green."

Bottom right: 1770: open-end extendable temples were a practical innovation. The 19th-century "clam shell case" shown is pressed steel covered with tin.

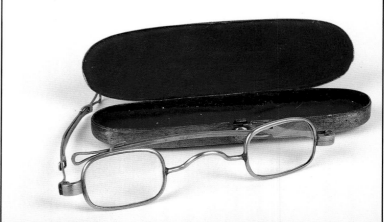

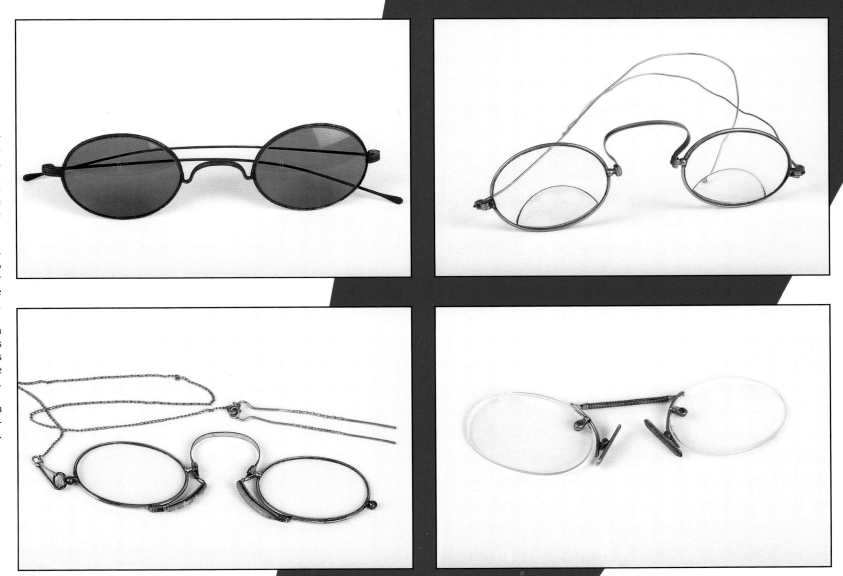

Top left: From 1871: an early "sun glass," with cobalt blue lenses. Colored lenses enjoyed a popularity resurrection after fashionable vampires donned them in the 1990s movie *Bram Stoker's Dracula*.

Top right: 1888: the "perfection bifocal" featured two pieces of glass joined together with a tongue-and-groove technique.

Bottom left: An innovation from 1890: this pince-nez has a hairpin at the end of its chain, eliminating necklace tangle.

Bottom right: Also from 1890: the bar spring pince-nez.

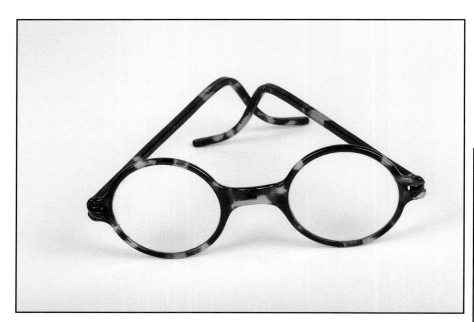

Enter the roaring '20s: during the Jazz Age of the 1920s, film comedian Harold Lloyd popularized spectacles with plastic frames.

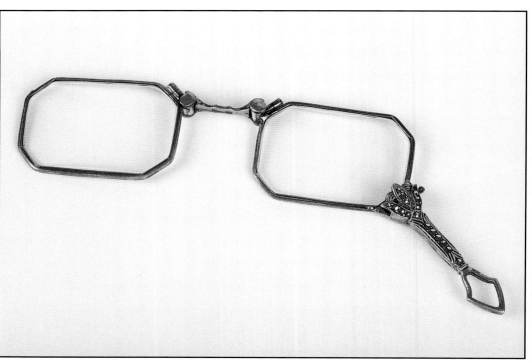

Circa 1930s: a "rhinestone" (marcasite) lorgnette.

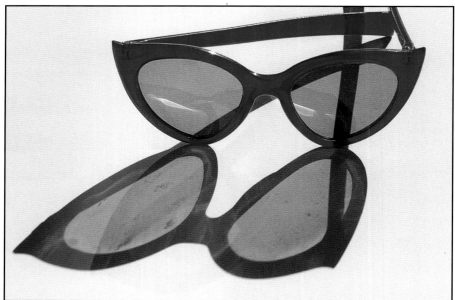

Also from the 1930s: the lady sees red, courtesy of this Parisian pair. $100-125.

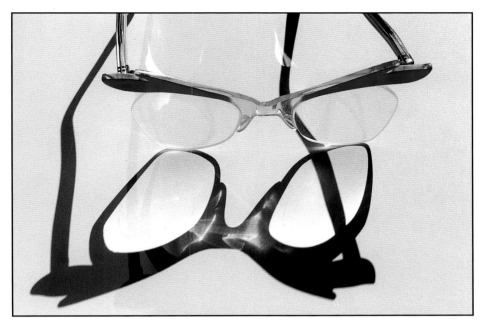

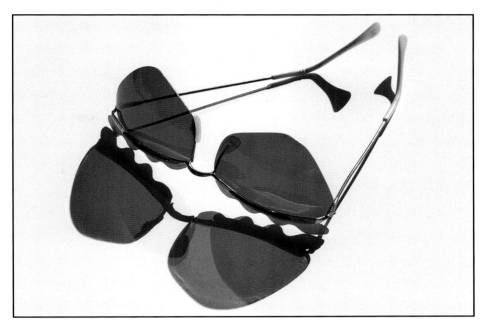

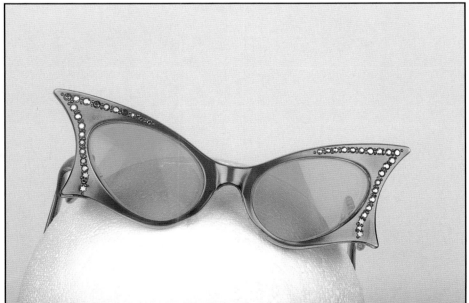

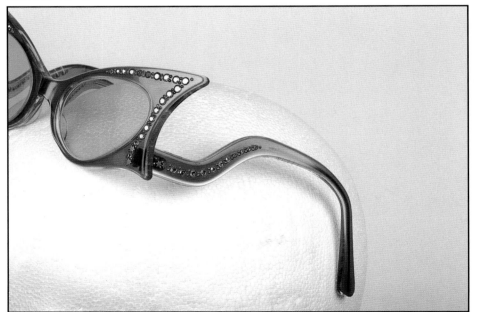

Top left: A '40s favorite: Ireland in the 1940s was the birthplace of this modernistic pair, with lenses suspended from a translucent painted frame. $100-125.

Top right: Another 1940s Dublin design: cobalt lenses with wire and ribbed plastic frame. $100-125.

Bottom left: The epitome of the fabulous '50s: double flare cat-eye frames in smoke with rhinestone decorations, yellow lenses. $140-160.

Bottom right: Temple detail.

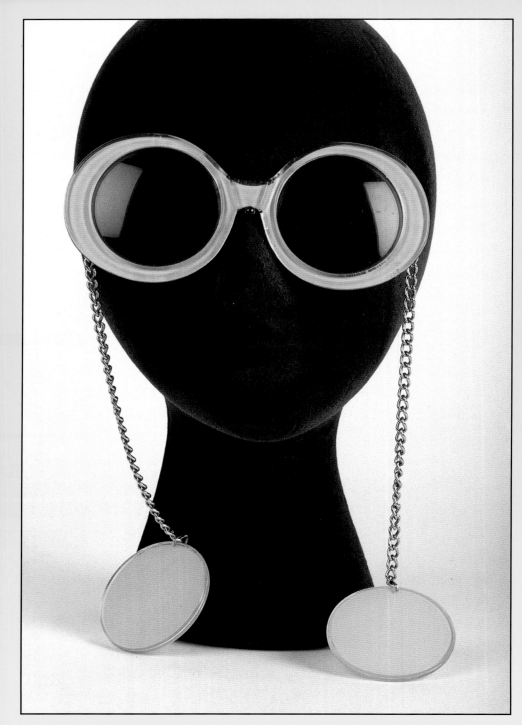

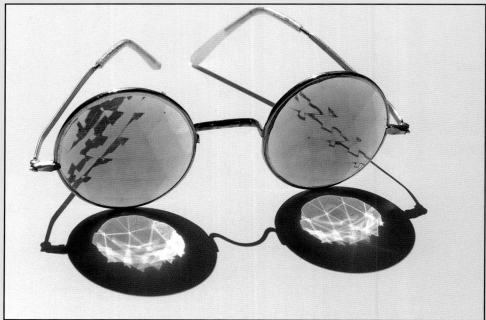

Direct from the 1960s: circular "hippie" frames with prismatic lenses. $60-75.

From the swinging '60s: circular op-art styling with "earring chains" replacing temples. It was an old idea revisited—medieval Chinese held their glasses in place with ear ribbons attached to weights. $120-160.

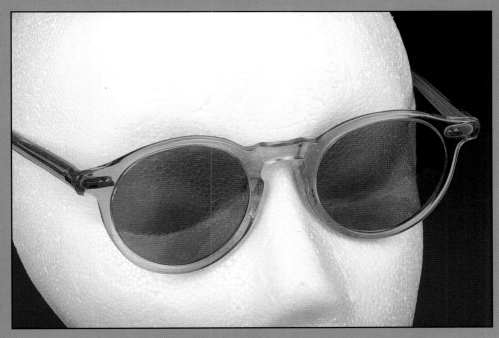

An authentic '70s souvenir: shades worn by Ramón Piña in 1971.

Bigger is better: from the 1970s, "Octette" by Selecta. The availability of larger lens blanks meant the possibility of larger frame styles. $50-60.

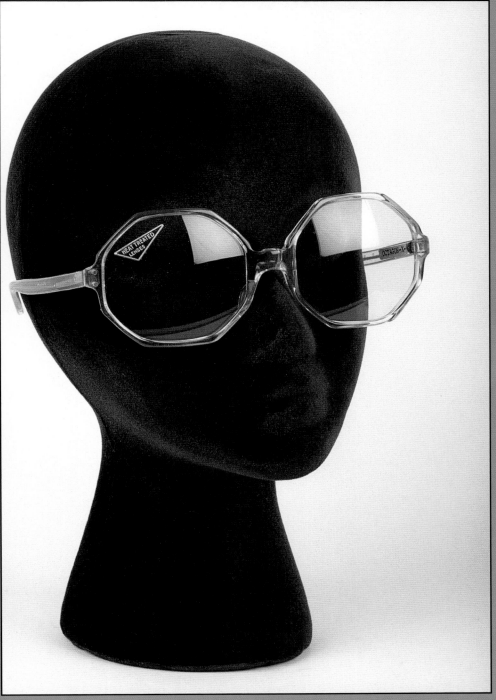

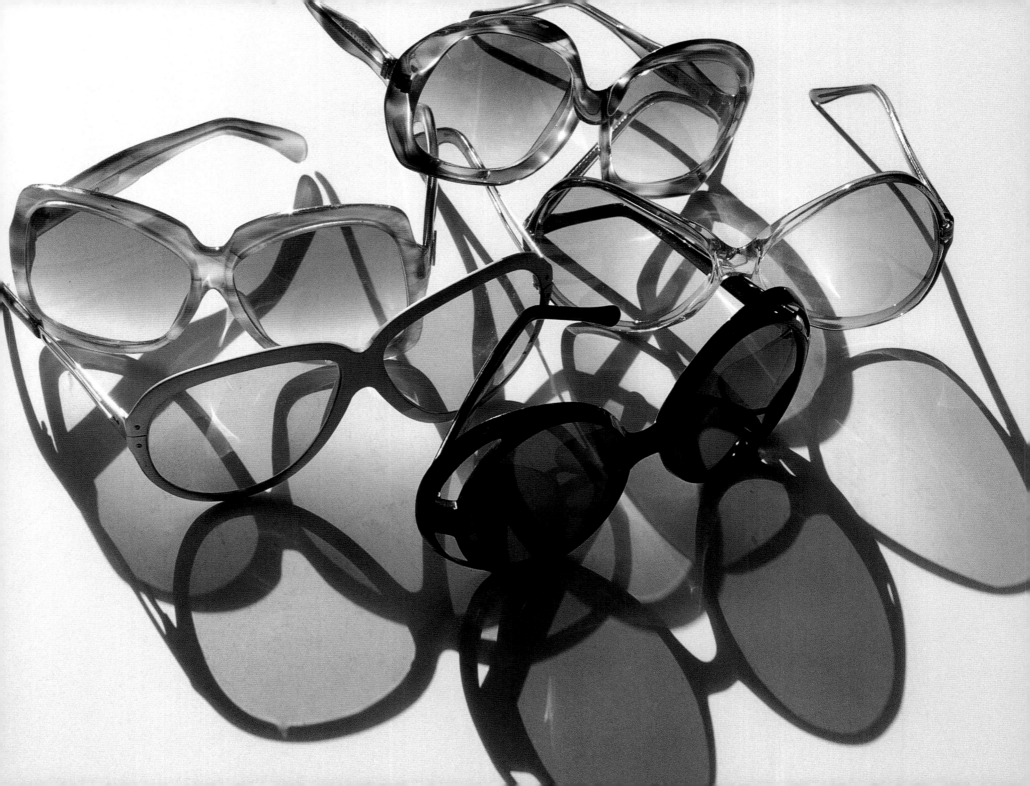

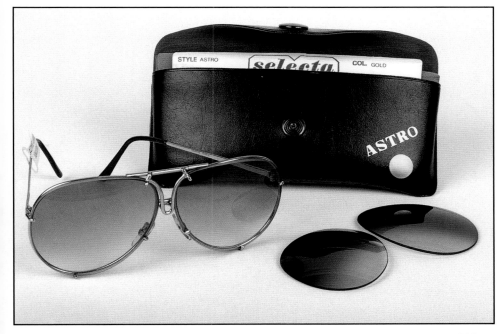

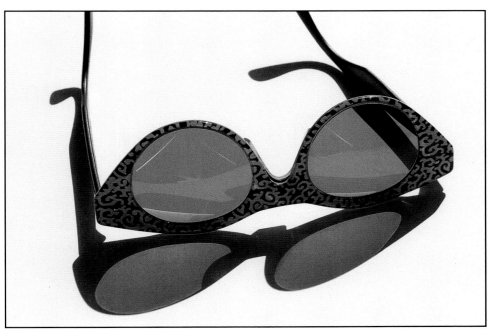

Aviator-style sun glasses, introduced in the 1930s, remained popular choices in the 1980s, as the decade embraced sports eyewear. This "Astro-Large Sporty Pilot Flip Up" model for men was introduced by Selecta in 1980. Exchangeable lenses were an extra selling point. $70-80.

The 1990s (or the 1930s, 1940s, and 1950s revisited!): sun glasses in a retro style. $40-50.

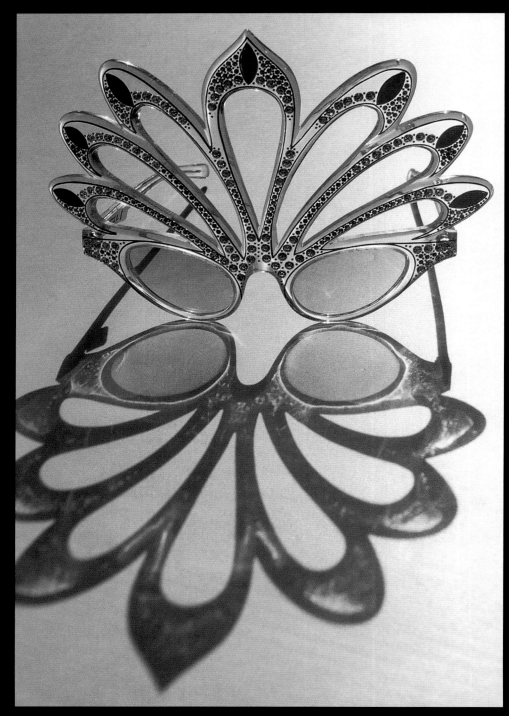

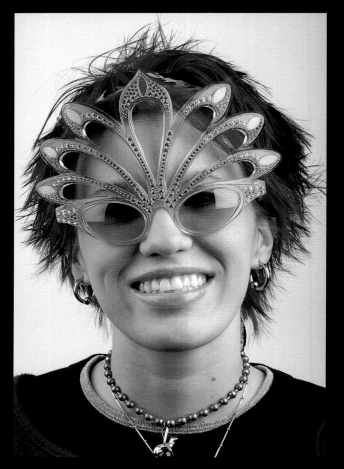

A modern "Miss Specs" models the highbrows.

Crowning achievement: elaborate highbrows distinguish this extravagant design, encompassing the best of every era. $1000-1200.

The beat goes on: another year, another "Miss Specs Appeal" (although for 1954 the winner was rechristened "Miss Beauty in Glasses"). The new titleholder, "startling blue-eyed blonde" Libby Booth, appeared as a guest on the Steve Allen TV show. Allen, "whose over-size specs are a trademark to thousands of viewers," listened attentively as Libby, a "vivacious Southern belle," related the importance of proper eyewear from both a visual and fashion point of view, and "demonstrated how various frames complemented her beauty." Then he got right to the point: "what an eyeful!"

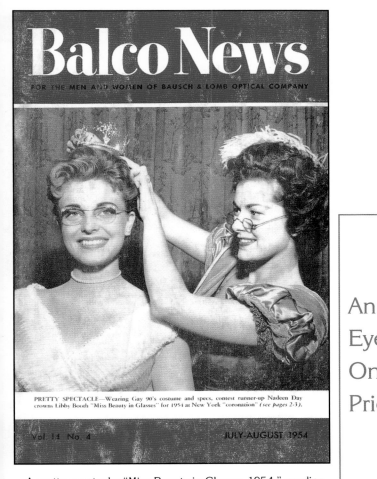

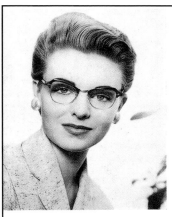

'The Eyes of Texas'

ONE GLANCE is enough to see why a board of judges picked 19-year-old Libby Booth (left) of Dallas, Tex., as the winner of this year's nation-wide Miss Beauty In Glasses Contest. A startling blue-eyed blonde, she's been wearing glasses for over nine years. The Balrims she's sporting offer conclusive proof to gals everywhere of just how effective proper eyewear can be in dramatizing a face.

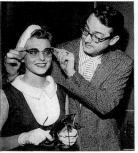

"WHAT AN EYEFUL," exclaims Steve Allen during Libby's New York appearance on his network TV show.

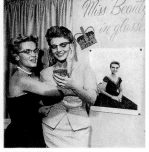

FAIR'S FAIREST—Adjusting Libby's Hi-Lite glasses at Chicago's Optical Fair is Nancy Ann Miller, 1953 winner.

Dallas Girl Reigns As 'Miss Beauty In Glasses'

IN NEWSREELS and newspapers, over television and radio, millions of people last month met America's most beautiful model who wears glasses.

A vivacious Southern belle and a real queen in every sense of the word, she's 19-year-old Libby Booth of Dallas, Tex. Winner of the second nation-wide "Miss Beauty in Glasses" competition, she was crowned queen at ceremonies in New York's Waldorf-Astoria Hotel.

At the "coronation," the first event in a mad, 10-day whirl of activities that included TV and radio appearances in New York and Rochester, were Fox-Movietone Newsreel cameramen, press photographers and fashion writers from several magazines. Also on hand, and

runner-up in the company-sponsored competition.

Before taking off two days later for the Optical Fair in Chicago, the petite, blue-eyed blonde appeared on the Steve Allen television show. Allen, whose over-size specs are a trademark to thousands of viewers, listened attentively as Libby related the importance of proper eyewear from both a visual and fashion point of view. "Modern frames for various occasions," she declared, "are as much a part of fashion today as shoes, hats, or jewelry."

At the Optical Fair in Chicago's Palmer House, ophthalmic customers by the hundred flocked to the Bausch & Lomb exhibit booth where Miss Beauty in

mer theatre group, modeled the new slate blue Hi-Lite frames, Balrims, Cordelle, Ray-Ban, and other B&L glasses.

Termed the "hit of the Fair" by Frame Sales manager Dick Eisenhart, she demonstrated how various frames complemented her beauty as well as the costumes furnished her by Dallas' famed Neiman-Marcus department store.

During her four-day visit to Rochester the following week, she toured the Lens plant, modeled for scores of photographs, appeared on a noon-hour show in the Main dining room, and was guest on three radio and TV programs.

"A real eyeful," Libby earned many times over the $300 in defense bonds she received for winning the contest.

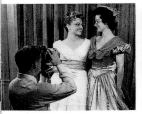

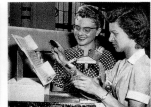

PRETTY SPECTACLE—Wearing Gay 90's costume and specs, contest runner-up Nadeen Day crowns Libby Booth "Miss Beauty in Glasses" for 1954 at New York "coronation" (see pages 2-3).

Vol. 14 No. 4   JULY-AUGUST 1954

A pretty spectacle: "Miss Beauty in Glasses 1954," exuding "specs appeal." (Her runner-up, the one in the granny glasses, exudes somewhat less!)

An Eye On Prices

Prices in *Specs Appeal* are based on glasses in mint to excellent condition. Ranges given are averages based on current selling prices and available information. As with any collectible, actual selling prices may vary with the locale or dealer. The suggested prices are most effective when used as a starting point to begin negotiations. While we cannot guarantee individual outcomes, we do guarantee you'll enjoy the view along the way!

Points to ponder:

* Broken lenses can always be replaced
* Metal frames can always be soldered.
* Plastic (or celluloid) frames cannot. If a frame is broken, purchase "for viewing purposes only." Without expert restoration, most damaged plastic frames cannot be cemented securely enough to provide the pressure necessary to hold a working lens.
* Temples, hinges, pads, and screws are almost always replaceable.
* The obvious restated: expect to pay more for the rare and the unique, including designer frames, unusual shapes (butterflies, birds, highbrows, and cat-eyes), and frames by such upscale manufacturers as Tura.
* "New Old Stock" (NOS) is always a great option. These are never-sold (and thus never-used) vintage frames, just waiting for your prescription!

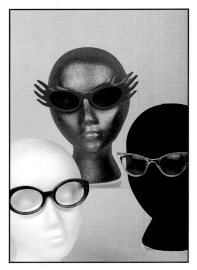

Chapter 2: "
THE EYES HAVE IT"

Eyewear For Everyday (And Night!)

Through a mock TV screen, salesmen previewed the continually expanding line of new frames and cases, in survey-tested new colors and trim. Then, with all the secrecy surrounding the unveiling of a new car, sales personnel enthusiastically endorsed the "Clubmaster," the "Spirelle," and the "Genesee."
— *Balco News*
March-April, 1955

Even the names are intoxicating: "Venus Pearl"—"Twilight Jewel"—"Sweetie Delight." As the "one pair is not enough" campaign caught fire in the '50s, the eyewear industry made the most of it. With only so many variations possible in the basic eyeglass shape, every additional sales point helped. Enticing model names were as important as keying certain eyewear styles to specific activities. Soon there were eye fashions for work, for play, for dress, and for everything in between. Something simple for a Sunday morning? "Balco Hi-Lites" were just right for church. Meeting for malts? Maybe "Coquette." Going "semi-casual?" Go for "Joselle." Or for a show-stopper, try "rhinestone-studded 'Cordelle' glasses for evening."

Included in this chapter are frames that suggest the range of fashion available in 1950s and '60s everyday and evening wear. Among the manufacturers represented are industry stalwarts American Optical, Art-Craft, B & L, Gandy, Hasday, Kono, Swank, Tura, Trans-World Eyewear Corporation (TWEC/TWE), and Victory. Also included are children's glasses (for the most part, junior adaptations of adult styles), men's, eyewear imports, laminates, and a selection of designer frames from such names as Christian Dior, Oleg Cassini, and Schiaparelli.

These are the glasses most commonly found by today's collectors; because they were produced in such volume, they are also among the most affordable. Fortunately, eyewear professionals can often install modern lenses in vintage frames. However, before snapping up the first pair that catches your fancy, a few items ("eye"-tems?) to consider:

• When trying on glasses, look your best. That way, you'll see the frames at their most flattering.

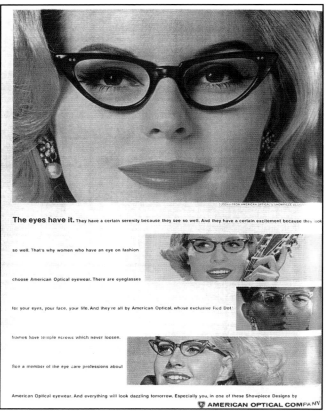

The eyes have it. They have a certain serenity because they see so well. And they have a certain excitement because they look

so well. That's why women who have an eye on fashion

choose American Optical eyewear. There are eyeglasses

for your eyes, your face, your life. And they're all by American Optical, whose exclusive Red Dot

frames have temple screws which never loosen.

See a member of the eye care professions about

American Optical eyewear. And everything will look dazzling tomorrow. Especially you, in one of these Showpiece Designs by

Ⓐ **AMERICAN OPTICAL COMPANY**

"The eyes have it: eyeglasses for your eyes, your face, your life." In the 1950s and '60s, consumers were urged to purchase glasses that provided an accurate reflection of their ever-changing personal style. If that meant more than one pair of glasses per customer, so much the better! This American Optical Company ad, which appeared in the July, 1965 issue of *Vogue*, promised "everything will look dazzling tomorrow. Especially you."

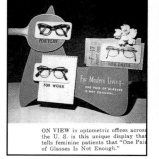

ON VIEW in optometric offices across the U. S. is this unique display that tells feminine patients that "One Pair of Glasses Is Not Enough."

As usual, Bausch & Lomb got there first. A 1955 promotional campaign reminded buyers that "One Pair of Glasses Is Not Enough." Who could be content without separate pairs "for work—for dress—for play?"

• Metals can almost always be adjusted, plastics can't. Make sure vintage plastic frames are a comfortable fit. Does the bridge rest easily on your nose? Are eyes centered? If not, and you plan on wearing them regularly, you may regret it.
• If you wear bifocals, opt for larger frames.
• If the temples are fancy, don't let your hair hide them.
• Bold frames call for big eyes and bold features. If yours aren't, eye makeup can help.
• Take your time, try on whatever seems appealing, and ask for opinions. Vintage frames are an investment. Invest wisely.
• Always remember: even in the '50s, cat-eyes weren't for everyone.

With a little practice (and a lot of shopping) you, like "Miss Specs Appeal," will soon be changing your eyewear as often as your earrings. Enjoy the sights!

BEAUTY IN GLASSES

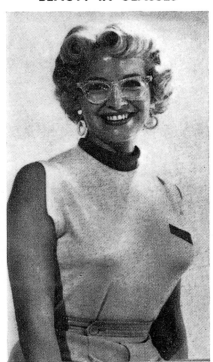

MOVIE STAR Marilyn Maxwell has joined the long list of glamour gals who agree it's time to bury **Dorothy Parker's** old couplet that "Men seldom make passes at girls who wear glasses."

In a national newspaper column, **Bob Thomas** *Associated Press* writer, points out that Marilyn not only wears glasses almost constantly, but keeps four pairs on hand for various activities. The pretty blonde even posed for cheesecake photos to prove that glasses don't detract from a girl's attraction. "I wear them wherever I go," she remarked, "and they've never seemed to stop men from making passes."

Marilyn admits she once tried to get by without glasses but "it didn't work. I walked into doors, tripped over curbs, and worst of all, I would walk right past my friends."

When word got back to her that she was snubbing her pals and offending bosses, she said to heck with glamour and put her spectacles back on. The consensus of opinion is that it hasn't hurt her glamour one bit *(AP photo)*.

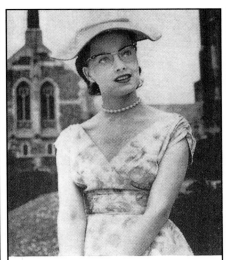

A VISION of loveliness, "Miss Beauty in Glasses" for 1955 favors Balco Hi-Lite frames for church, formal wear.

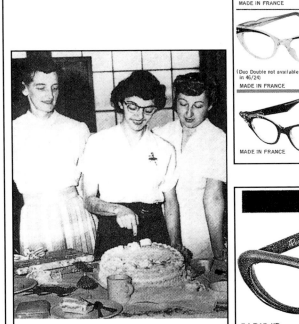

BRIDE-TO-BE Carmela Silvestri, Navy Building, cuts cake at a gift-laden shower given by gals in N-11.

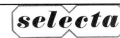
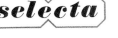
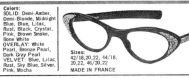

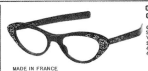
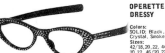
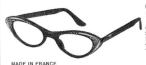
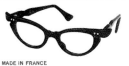
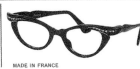
Left: Manufacturers worked overtime to dispel the "glasses stigma" of bygone days. B & L celebrity spokesperson Marilyn Maxwell kept "four pairs on hand for various activities." The va-va-voom movie gal "even posed for cheesecake photos to prove that glasses don't detract from a girl's attraction." So there!

Top center: Proving the point, here's "Miss Beauty in Glasses 1955" modeling a new B & L frame.

Bottom center: Did it work for regular girls? You be the judge.

Top right: Some '50s styles had staying power. Although "cat-eye" frames first attained popularity in the 1950s, this selection from Selecta was featured in their 1980 catalog!

Bottom right: Find a frame you like, but too dressy (or not dressy enough) for all occasions? No problem. As this "Paris" illustration indicates, most frames were available in both plain and decorative styles.

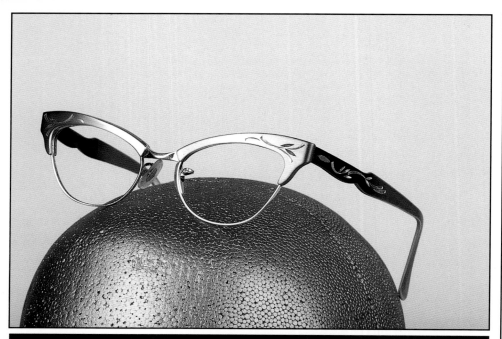

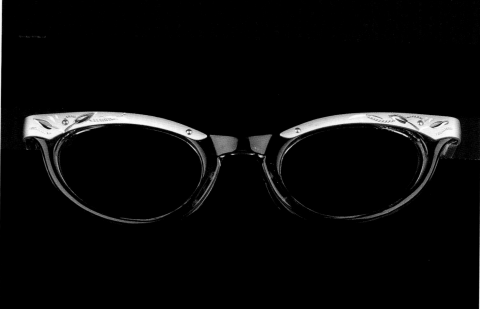

Top: By American Optical: brown frames with aluminum brows and temples. $50-60.

Bottom: A similar American Optical in smoke. $50-60.

AMERICAN OPTICAL CO.

MAY MFG. CORP.

ART-CRAFT

ART-CRAFT CO., INC.

George E. Koch Inc.
P.O. BOX 377, PLANETARIUM STATION
NEW YORK, NEW YORK 10024
2315 BROADWAY   (212) 787-3355

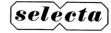

BAUSCH & LOMB ▼
Mark of Leadership

BAUSCH & LOMB, INC.

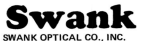

SHURON CONTINENTAL

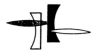

GOTHAM OPTICAL CO., INC.

Swank
SWANK OPTICAL CO., INC.

GRACELINE

TRANS-WORLD EYEWEAR

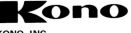

KONO, INC.

TURA, INC.

MARINE OPTICAL MFG. CO.

Victory Optical

VICTORY OPTICAL MFG. CO.,
INC.

Wondering who made what? Here are some of the most popular eyewear manufacturers of the 1950s and '60s, along with their corporate symbols, often used as eyeglass identifiers.

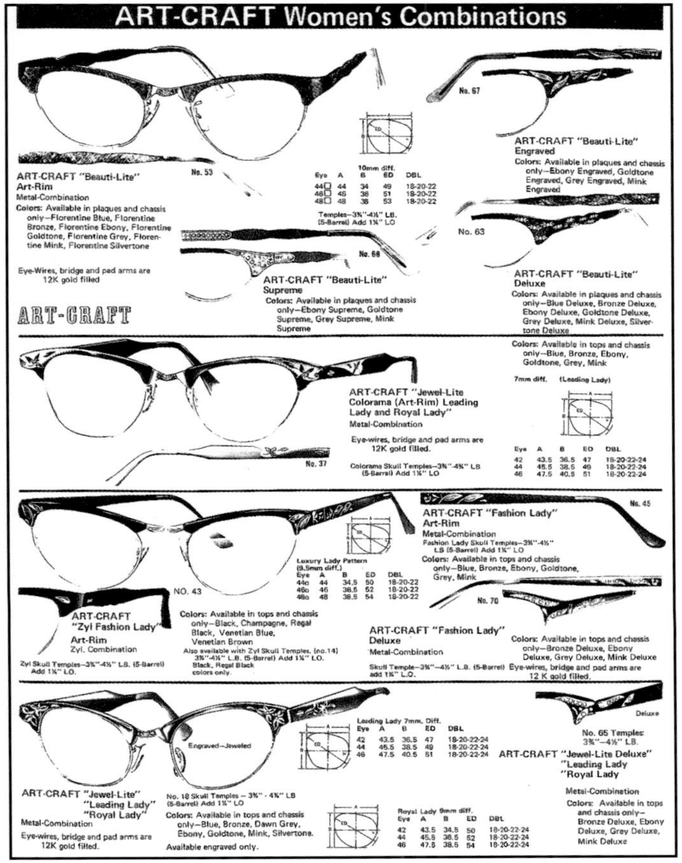

ART-CRAFT Women's Combinations

No. 53

ART-CRAFT "Beauti-Lite" Art-Rim
Metal-Combination
Colors: Available in plaques and chassis only—Florentine Blue, Florentine Bronze, Florentine Ebony, Florentine Goldtone, Florentine Grey, Florentine Mink, Florentine Silvertone

Eye-Wires, bridge and pad arms are 12K gold filled

Eye	A	B (10mm diff.)	ED	DBL
44☐	44	34	49	18-20-22
46☐	46	36	51	18-20-22
48☐	48	38	53	18-20-22

Temples—3¾"-4½" LB. (5-Barrel) Add 1¼" LO

No. 67

ART-CRAFT "Beauti-Lite" Engraved
Colors: Available in plaques and chassis only—Ebony Engraved, Goldtone Engraved, Grey Engraved, Mink Engraved

No. 68

ART-CRAFT "Beauti-Lite" Supreme
Colors: Available in plaques and chassis only—Ebony Supreme, Goldtone Supreme, Grey Supreme, Mink Supreme

No. 63

ART-CRAFT "Beauti-Lite" Deluxe
Colors: Available in plaques and chassis only—Blue Deluxe, Bronze Deluxe, Ebony Deluxe, Goldtone Deluxe, Grey Deluxe, Mink Deluxe, Silvertone Deluxe

ART-CRAFT

No. 37

ART-CRAFT "Jewel-Lite Colorama (Art-Rim) Leading Lady and Royal Lady"
Metal-Combination
Eye-wires, bridge and pad arms are 12K gold filled.
Colorama Skull Temples—3¾"-4¾" LB (5-Barrel) Add 1¼" LO

Colors: Available in tops and chassis only—Blue, Bronze, Ebony, Goldtone, Grey, Mink

7mm diff. (Leading Lady)

Eye	A	B	ED	DBL
42	43.5	36.5	47	18-20-22-24
44	45.5	38.5	49	18-20-22-24
46	47.5	40.5	51	18-20-22-24

NO. 43

Luxury Lady Pattern (9.5mm diff.)

Eye	A	B	ED	DBL
44o	44	34.5	50	18-20-22
46o	46	36.5	52	18-20-22
48o	48	38.5	54	18-20-22

No. 45

ART-CRAFT "Fashion Lady" Art-Rim
Metal-Combination
Fashion Lady Skull Temples—3¾"-4½" LB (5-Barrel) Add 1¼" LO
Colors: Available in tops and chassis only—Blue, Bronze, Ebony, Goldtone, Grey, Mink

ART-CRAFT "Zyl Fashion Lady" Art-Rim
Zyl. Combination
Zyl Skull Temples—3¾"-4½" L.B. (5-Barrel) Add 1¼" LO.

Colors: Available in tops and chassis only—Black, Champagne, Regal Black, Venetian Blue, Venetian Brown
Also available with Zyl Skull Temples, (no.14) 3¾"-4½" L.B. (5-Barrel) Add 1¼" LO. Black, Regal Black colors only.

No. 70

ART-CRAFT "Fashion Lady" Deluxe
Metal-Combination
Skull Temple—3¾"—4½" L.B. (5-Barrel) add 1¼" L.O.

Colors: Available in tops and chassis only—Bronze Deluxe, Ebony Deluxe, Grey Deluxe, Mink Deluxe
Eye-wires, bridge and pad arms are 12 K gold filled.

Engraved—Jeweled

ART-CRAFT "Jewel-Lite" "Leading Lady" "Royal Lady"
Metal-Combination
Eye-wires, bridge and pad arms are 12K gold filled.

No. 18 Skull Temples – 3¾" - 4¾" LB (5-Barrel) Add 1¼" LO
Colors: Available in tops and chassis only—Blue, Bronze, Dawn Grey, Ebony, Goldtone, Mink, Silvertone.
Available engraved only.

Leading Lady 7mm. Diff.

Eye	A	B	ED	DBL
42	43.5	36.5	47	18-20-22-24
44	45.5	38.5	49	18-20-22-24
46	47.5	40.5	51	18-20-22-24

Royal Lady 9mm diff.

Eye	A	B	ED	DBL
42	43.5	34.5	50	18-20-22-24
44	45.5	36.5	52	18-20-22-24
46	47.5	38.5	54	18-20-22-24

Deluxe

No. 65 Temples: 3¾"—4½" LB.

ART-CRAFT "Jewel-Lite Deluxe" "Leading Lady "Royal Lady
Metal-Combination
Colors: Available in tops and chassis only—Bronze Deluxe, Ebony Deluxe, Grey Deluxe, Mink Deluxe

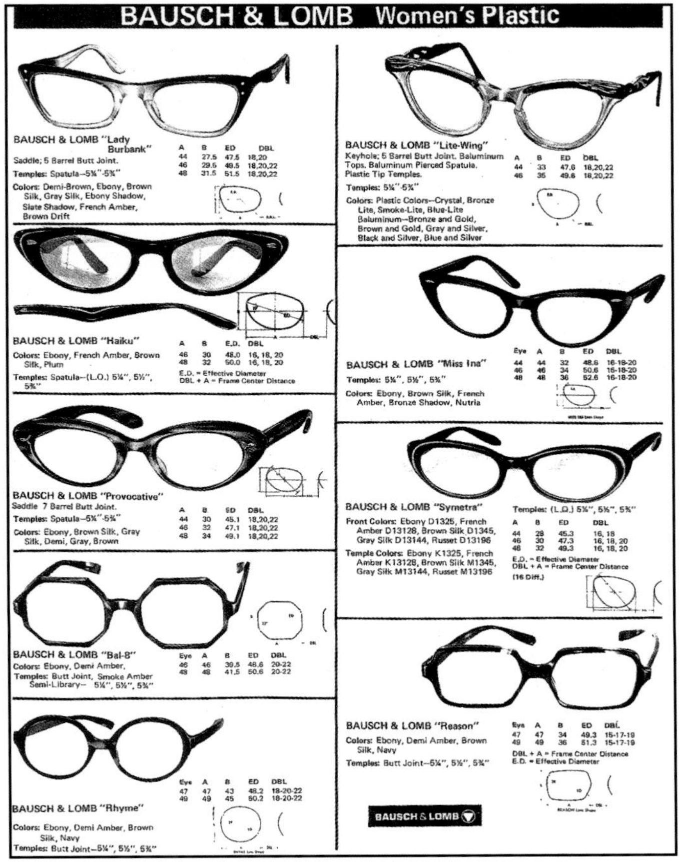

BAUSCH & LOMB Women's Plastic

BAUSCH & LOMB "Lady Burbank"
Saddle; 5 Barrel Butt Joint.
Temples: Spatula—5¼"-5¾"
Colors: Demi-Brown, Ebony, Brown Silk, Gray Silk, Ebony Shadow, Slate Shadow, French Amber, Brown Drift

A	B	ED	DBL
44	27.5	47.5	18,20
46	29.5	49.5	18,20,22
48	31.5	51.5	18,20,22

BAUSCH & LOMB "Haiku"
Colors: Ebony, French Amber, Brown Silk, Plum
Temples: Spatula—(L.O.) 5¼", 5½", 5¾"

A	B	E.D.	DBL
46	30	48.0	16, 18, 20
48	32	50.0	16, 18, 20

E.D. = Effective Diameter
DBL + A = Frame Center Distance

BAUSCH & LOMB "Provocative"
Saddle 7 Barrel Butt Joint.
Temples: Spatula—5¼"-5¾"
Colors: Ebony, Brown Silk, Gray Silk, Demi, Gray, Brown

A	B	ED	DBL
44	30	45.1	18,20,22
46	32	47.1	18,20,22
48	34	49.1	18,20,22

BAUSCH & LOMB "Bal-8"
Colors: Ebony, Demi Amber,
Temples: Butt Joint, Smoke Amber Semi-Library— 5¼", 5½", 5¾"

Eye	A	B	ED	DBL
46	46	39.5	48.6	20-22
48	48	41.5	50.6	20-22

Eye	A	B	ED	DBL
47	47	43	48.2	18-20-22
49	49	45	50.2	18-20-22

BAUSCH & LOMB "Rhyme"
Colors: Ebony, Demi Amber, Brown Silk, Navy
Temples: Butt Joint—5¼", 5½", 5¾"

BAUSCH & LOMB "Lite-Wing"
Keyhole; 5 Barrel Butt Joint, Baluminum Tops, Baluminum Pierced Spatula, Plastic Tip Temples.
Temples: 5¼"-5¾"
Colors: Plastic Colors—Crystal, Bronze Lite, Smoke-Lite, Blue-Lite Baluminum—Bronze and Gold, Brown and Gold, Gray and Silver, Black and Silver, Blue and Silver

A	B	ED	DBL
44	33	47.6	18,20,22
46	35	49.6	18,20,22

BAUSCH & LOMB "Miss Ina"
Temples: 5¼", 5½", 5¾"
Colors: Ebony, Brown Silk, French Amber, Bronze Shadow, Nutria

Eye	A	B	ED	DBL
44	44	32	48.6	16-18-20
46	46	34	50.6	16-18-20
48	48	36	52.6	16-18-20

BAUSCH & LOMB "Symetra"
Front Colors: Ebony D1325, French Amber D13128, Brown Silk D1345, Gray Silk D13144, Russet D13196
Temple Colors: Ebony K1325, French Amber K13128, Brown Silk M1345, Gray Silk M13144, Russet M13196
Temples: (L.O.) 5¼", 5½", 5¾"

A	B	ED	DBL
44	28	45.3	16, 18
46	30	47.3	16, 18, 20
48	32	49.3	16, 18, 20

E.D. = Effective Diameter
DBL + A = Frame Center Distance
(16 Diff.)

BAUSCH & LOMB "Reason"
Colors: Ebony, Demi Amber, Brown Silk, Navy
Temples: Butt Joint—5¼", 5½", 5¾"

Eye	A	B	ED	DBL
47	47	34	49.3	15-17-19
49	49	36	51.3	15-17-19

DBL + A = Frame Center Distance
E.D. = Effective Diameter

BAUSCH & LOMB

Top left: Stylings by Art-Craft.

Bottom left: Aluminum combinations by Art-Craft, in silver with rhinestone decoration. $50-60.

Top right: Frames by Bausch & Lomb.

Bottom: 1955 B & L favorites, the "Hi-Lites" and "Joselle."

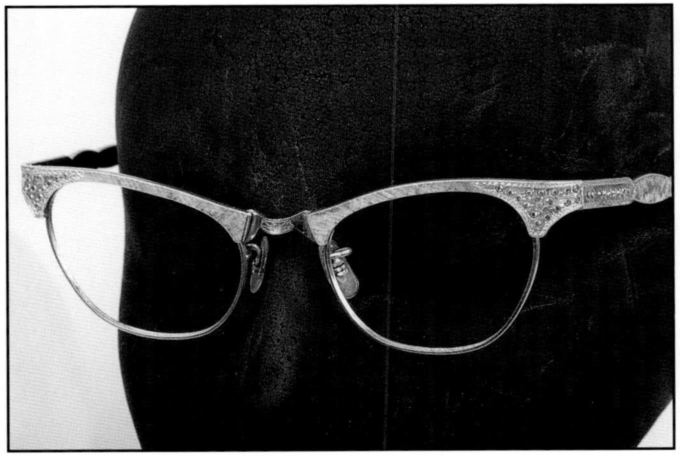

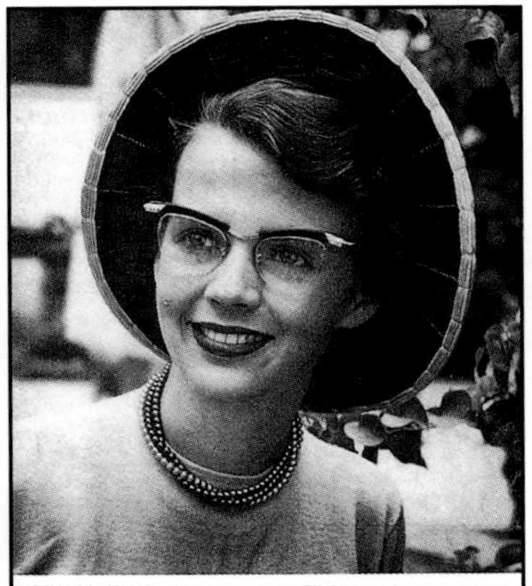

SPEC-TACULAR—The new ebony Hi-Lite with wrap-around trim, was the popular hit of a recent Palm Beach fashion show.

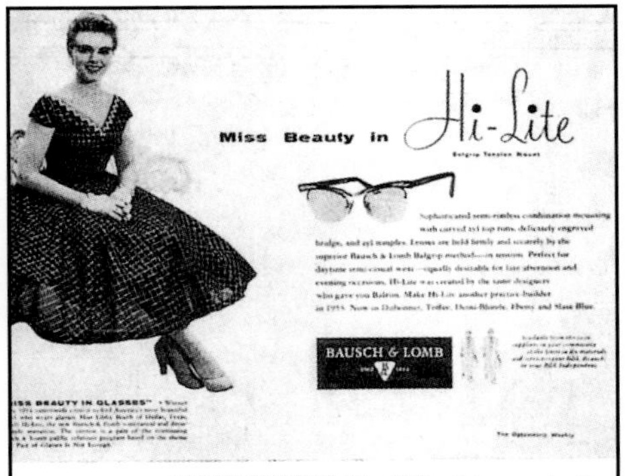

CENTERSPREAD ADS, this one in the *Optometric Weekly*, feature the new Hi-Lite mounting. The model is Miss Libby Booth, "Miss Beauty in Glasses" of 1954.

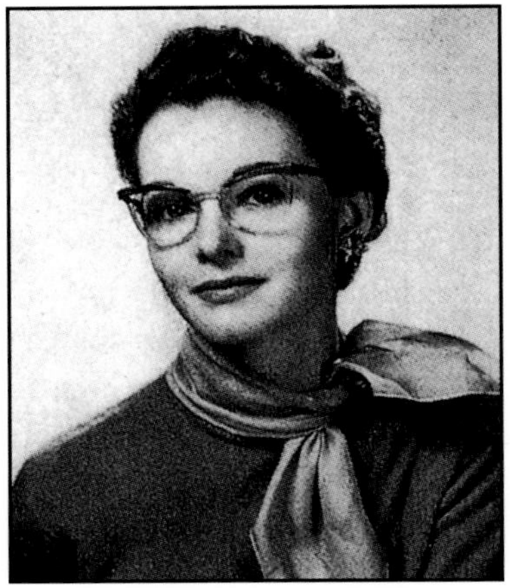

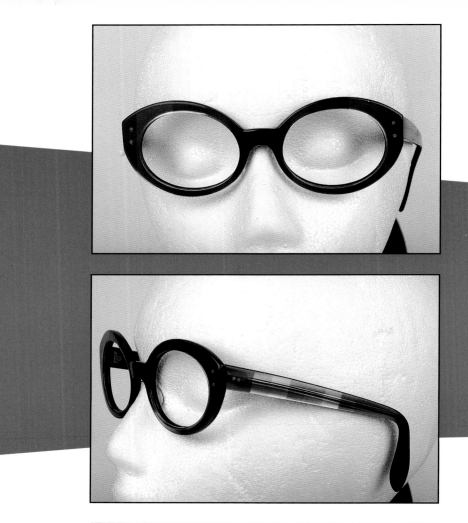

Top: "Bewitching" by Bausch & Lomb. $70-85.

Center: Detail, "Bewitching's" rainbow temple.

Bottom: Smokey ovals by B & L, in the shape often referred to as "Jackie O's." $60-70.

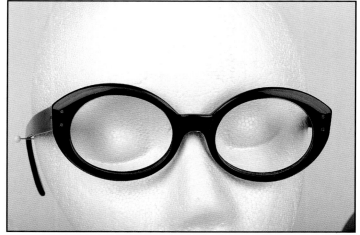

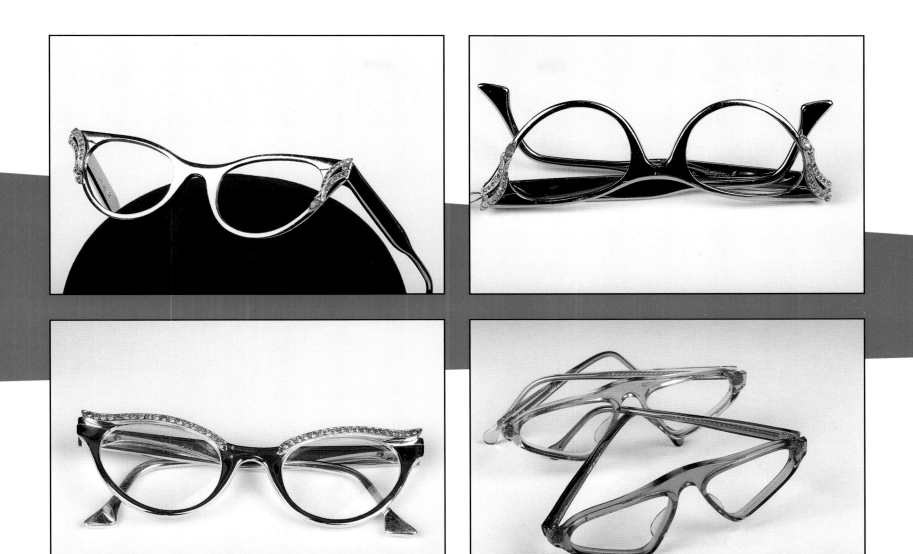

Top left: By J. Hasday, silver-grey frames with rhinestone swags at brow edge. $70-85.

Top right: Detail.

Bottom left: Also by J. Hasday, silver with rhinestone brows. $70-85.

Bottom right: Made in Italy for Gandy, unique "point" frames in smoke and tan. $45-55 each.

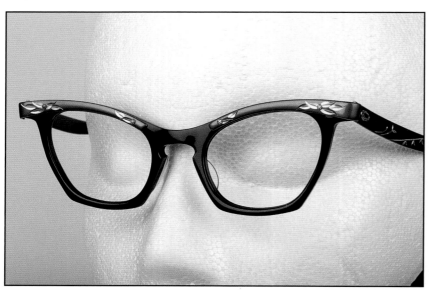

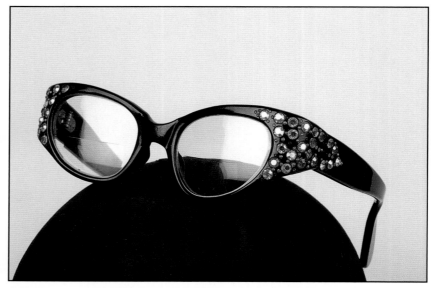

KONO Women's Zyl

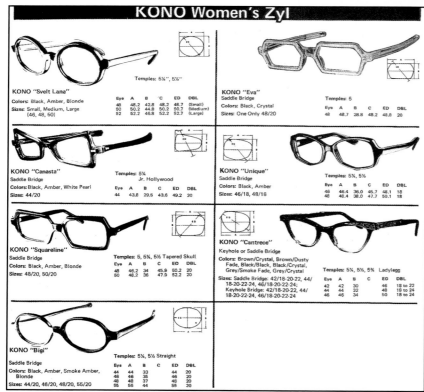

KONO "Svelt Lana"
Colors: Black, Amber, Blonde
Sizes: Small, Medium, Large
(46, 48, 50)

Temples: 5¼", 5½"

Eye	A	B	C	ED	DBL	
48	48.2	42.8	48.2	48.7	(Small)
50	50.2	44.8	50.2	50.7	(Medium)
52	52.2	46.8	52.2	52.7	(Large)

KONO "Eva"
Saddle Bridge
Colors: Black, Crystal
Sizes: One Only 48/20

Temples: 5

Eye	A	B	C	ED	DBL
48	48.7	28.8	48.2	48.8	20

KONO "Canasta"
Saddle Bridge
Colors: Black, Amber, White Pearl
Sizes: 44/20

Temples: 5¼
Jr. Hollywood

Eye	A	B	C	ED	DBL
44	43.8	29.5	43.6	49.2	20

KONO "Unique"
Saddle Bridge
Colors: Black, Amber
Sizes: 46/18, 48/18

Temples: 5¼, 5½

Eye	A	B	C	ED	DBL
46	46.4	36.0	45.7	48.1	18
48	48.4	38.0	47.7	50.1	18

KONO "Squareline"
Saddle Bridge
Colors: Black, Amber, Blonde
Sizes: 48/20, 50/20

Temples: 5, 5¼, 5½ Tapered Skull

Eye	A	B	C	ED	DBL
48	46.2	34	45.9	50.2	20
50	48.2	36	47.9	52.2	20

KONO "Cantrece"
Keyhole or Saddle Bridge
Colors: Brown/Crystal, Brown/Dusty
Fade, Black/Black, Black/Crystal,
Grey/Smoke Fade, Grey/Crystal

Sizes: Saddle Bridge: 42/18-20-22, 44/
18-20-22-24, 46/18-20-22-24;
Keyhole Bridge: 42/18-20-22, 44/
18-20-22-24, 46/18-20-22-24

Temples: 5¼, 5½, 5¾ Ladylegg

Eye	A	B	C	ED	DBL
42	42	30	46	18 to 22
44	44	32	48	18 to 24
46	46	34	50	18 to 24

KONO "Bigi"
Saddle Bridge
Colors: Black, Amber, Smoke Amber,
Blonde
Sizes: 44/20, 46/20, 48/20, 55/20

Temples: 5¼, 5½ Straight

Eye	A	B	C	ED	DBL
44	44	33	44	20
46	46	35	46	20
48	48	37	48	20
55	56	44	55	20

SWANK Women's Zyl

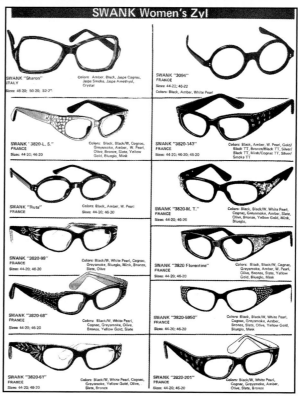

SWANK "Sharon"
ITALY
Sizes: 48-20; 50-20; 52-2"
Colors: Amber, Black, Jaspe Cognac,
Jaspe Smoke, Jaspe Amethyst,
Crystal

SWANK "3094"
FRANCE
Sizes: 44-22; 46-22
Colors: Black, Amber, White Pearl

SWANK "3820-L. S."
FRANCE
Sizes: 44-20; 46-20
Colors: Black, Black/W, Cognac,
Greysmoke, Amber, W. Pearl,
Olive, Bronze, Slate, Yellow
Gold, Blueglo, Mink

SWANK "3820-143"
FRANCE
Sizes: 44-20; 46-20; 48-20
Colors: Black, Amber, W. Pearl, Gold/
Black TT, Bronze/Black TT, Silver/
Black TT, Mismk/Cognac TT, Silver/
Smoke TT

SWANK "Ruta"
FRANCE
Sizes: 44-20; 46-20
Colors: Black, Amber, W. Pearl

SWANK "3820-M. T."
FRANCE
Sizes: 44-20; 46-20
Colors: Black, Black/W, White Pearl,
Cognac, Greysmoke, Amber, Slate,
Olive, Bronze, Yellow Gold, Mink,
Blueglo

SWANK "3820-99"
FRANCE
Sizes: 44-20; 46-20
Colors: Black/W, White Pearl, Cognac,
Greysmoke, Blueglo, Mink, Bronze,
Slate, Olive

SWANK "3820 Florentine"
FRANCE
Sizes: 44-20; 46-20
Colors: Black, Black/W, White Pearl,
Greysmoke, Amber, W. Pearl,
Olive, Bronze, Slate, Yellow
Gold, Blueglo, Mink

SWANK "3820-68"
FRANCE
Sizes: 44-20; 46-20
Colors: Black/W, White Pearl,
Cognac, Greysmoke, Olive,
Bronze, Yellow Gold, Slate

SWANK "3820-5950"
FRANCE
Sizes: 44-20; 46-20
Colors: Black, Black/W, White Pearl,
Cognac, Greysmoke, Amber,
Bronze, Slate, Olive, Yellow Gold,
Blueglo, Olive

SWANK "3820-61"
FRANCE
Sizes: 44-20; 46-20
Colors: Black/W, White Pearl, Cognac,
Greysmoke, Yellow Gold, Olive,
Slate, Bronze

SWANK "3820-201"
FRANCE
Sizes: 44-20; 46-20
Colors: Black/W, White Pearl, Cognac,
Greysmoke, Amber,
Olive, Slate, Bronze

Top left: From Kono, aluminum combinations in black with steel blue decorated brow. $55-65.

Bottom left: Frame selections by Kono.

Top right: Swank's "3820-L.S." in black with oversize rhinestones. $130-150.

Bottom right: A selection of frames for women by Swank.

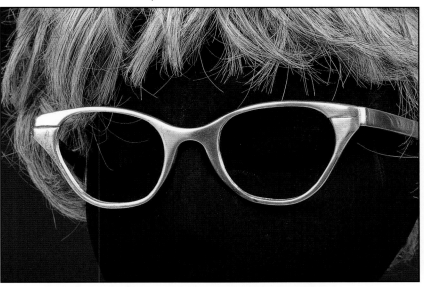

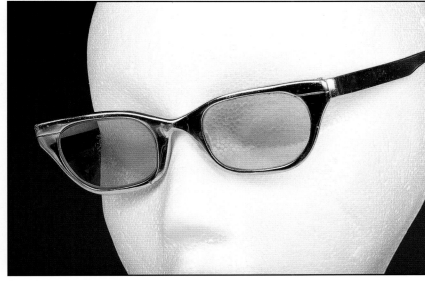

Top left: An unadorned Tura frame in plain silver. $60-70.

Top right: The same frame in plain gold—with green lenses! $70-80

Bottom left and right: Frame fashions by Tura, "the Cadillac of eyewear."

TURA Women's Frames

"Q" SHAPE	"Q" Shape: 110 difference—44/20, 44/22, 46/20
	Multi-fit interchangeable plastic pads and rocking pads available.
	Basic Frame Colors: Satin Ebony Satin Mink Satin Bronze
	  Satin Silver Satin Oxford Pearl
	Fashion Frame Colors:
	  Satin Pink Satin Green
	  Satin Silver Satin Blue
	Temples: Style "B"—vinyl tipped 5½, 5¾, 6" Shiny Gold (After 5)

"T" SHAPE	"T" Shape: (14 difference—46/20, 46/22 Multi-fit plastic pads and rocking pads are available. Colors: Only available in Satin Ebony, Satin Mink, Satin Bronze, Pearl, Satin Silver, and After Five (Shiny Gold Color)

Tura

TURA "Plain"
Shape: "Q" and "T"
Sizes: All sizes in each shape
Colors: All 10 colors of the "Q" shape
All 6 colors of the "T" shape

TURA "Flirtation Engraving"
Shape: "Q" shape and "T" shape
NOTE: This engraved Flirtation design is the only engraved design available in the women's "T" shape and the only engraved design available in ALL colors of the "Q" shape.
Sizes: All
Colors: All colors of the "Q" shape
All colors of the "T" shape
NOTE: Although this appears to be a jeweled design, there are no stones. The effect is created by the hand engraving.

TURA "No. 70 Engraving"
Gold color engraving with Silver Stars
Shape: "Q" shape ONLY
Sizes: ALL
Colors: Only in Satin Bronze, Satin Mink, Satin Ebony, Satin Silver. For an engraved design in shiny frame colors see the "Flirtation Engraving".

TURA "No. 303"
Gives the beauty effect of slenderizing the broad bridge.
Shape: "Q" shape ONLY
Sizes: ALL
Colors: All frame colors with Gold or Silver color design.

TURA "No. 307"
Shape: "Q" shape and "T" shape
Sizes: ALL
Colors: All 10 colors of the "Q" shape
All 6 colors of the "T" shape. Gold or Silver color design.

TURA "No. 308"
Gives the beauty effect of slenderizing a full face.
Shape: "Q" shape only
Sizes: ALL
Colors: All frame colors of the "Q" shape. Gold or Silver color design.

TURA "No. 257"
Two-tone Gold and Silver color Filigree design.
Shape: "Q" shape and "T" shape
Sizes: ALL
Colors: All 10 colors of the "Q" shape
All 6 colors of the "T" shape.

TURA "Filigree Design No. 657"
Two-tone gold and silver color filigree design. On front and temples.
Shape: "Q" shape and "T" shape
Sizes: ALL
Colors: All colors of the "Q" shape
All colors of the "T" shape

TURA "Jeweled No. 720"
2-tone gold and silver color design with 16-cultured pearls or genuine tiger eye agate.
Shape: "Q" shape and "T" shape
Sizes: ALL
Colors: All 10 colors of the "Q" shape
All 6 colors of the "T" shape
Available with white cultured pearls or brown tiger eye agate.

TURA "The Exclusive"
This design is normally on front and temples. Photo shows design on front only.
Shape: "Q" shape and "T" shape
Sizes: ALL
Colors: All 17 colors of the "Q" shape
All 5 colors of the "T" shape

TURA "No. 702 Strictly Private"
Shape: "Q" shape and "T" shape
Sizes: ALL
Colors: All 10 colors of the "Q" shape
All 6 colors of the "T" shape
Available in following combinations:
STONES
Pearls and Clear Navettes
DESIGN COLOR
Silver or Gold
Round crystals and topaz, Navettes (no pearls) Gold only
Round crystals and Sapphires, Navettes (no pearls) Silver only
Round crystals and Black, Navettes (no pearls) Silver only

TURA "No. 703"
Shape: "Q" shape and "T" shape
Sizes: ALL
Colors: All 10 colors of the "Q" shape
All 6 colors of the "T" shape
Front and temple design in either Gold or Silver depending upon frame color.
16 cultured pearls.

TURA "No. 704"
Shape: "Q" shape and "T" shape
Sizes: ALL
Colors: All 10 colors of the "Q" shape
All 6 colors of the "T" shape
Front and temple design in either Gold or Silver depending upon frame color.
20 cultured pearls.

TURA Women's Frames

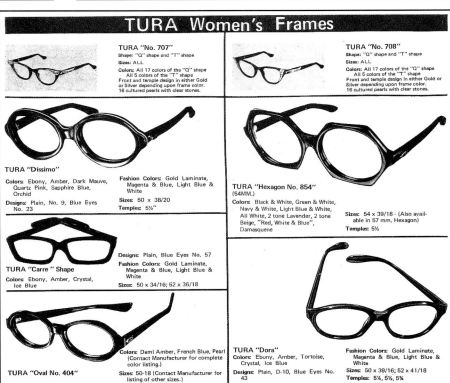

TURA "No. 707"
Shape: "Q" shape and "T" shape
Sizes: ALL.
Colors: All 17 colors of the "Q" shape
All 5 colors of the "T" shape
Front and temple design in either Gold or Silver depending upon frame color.
16 cultured pearls with clear stones.

TURA "No. 708"
Shape: "Q" shape and "T" shape
Sizes: ALL.
Colors: All 17 colors of the "Q" shape
All 5 colors of the "T" shape
Front and temple design in either Gold or Silver depending upon frame color.
16 cultured pearls with clear stones.

TURA "Dissimo"
Colors: Ebony, Amber, Dark Mauve, Quartz Pink, Sapphire Blue, Orchid
Designs: Plain, No. 9, Blue Eyes No. 23
Fashion Colors: Gold Laminate, Magenta & Blue, Light Blue & White
Sizes: 50 x 38/20
Temples: 5½"

TURA "Hexagon No. 854"
(54MM.)
Colors: Black & White, Green & White, Navy & White, Light Blue & White, All White, 2 tone Lavender, 2 tone Beige, "Red, White & Blue", Damasquene
Sizes: 54 x 39/18 - (Also available in 57 mm. Hexagon)
Temples: 5½

TURA "Carre" Shape
Colors: Ebony, Amber, Crystal, Ice Blue
Designs: Plain, Blue Eyes No. 57
Fashion Colors: Gold Laminate, Magenta & Blue, Light Blue & White
Sizes: 50 x 34/16; 52 x 36/18

TURA "Oval No. 404"
Colors: Demi Amber, French Blue, Pearl (Contact Manufacturer for complete color listing.)
Sizes: 50-18 (Contact Manufacturer for listing of other sizes.)

TURA "Dora"
Colors: Ebony, Amber, Tortoise, Crystal, Ice Blue
Designs: Plain, D-10, Blue Eyes No. 43
Fashion Colors: Gold Laminate, Magenta & Blue, Light Blue & White
Sizes: 50 x 39/16; 52 x 41/18
Temples: 5¼, 5½, 5¾

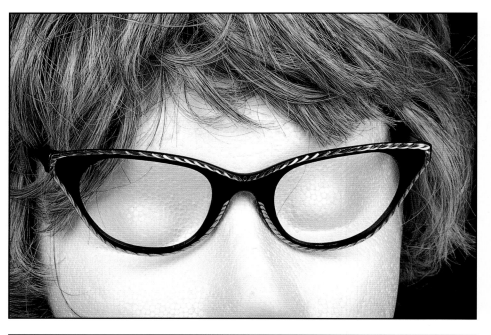

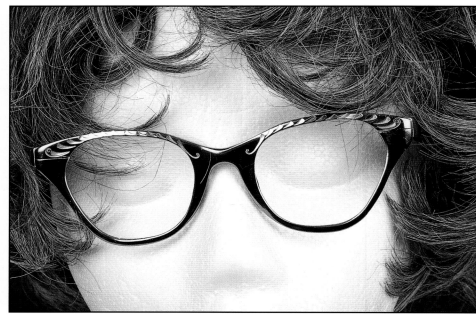

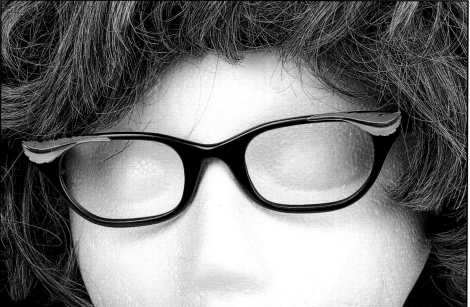

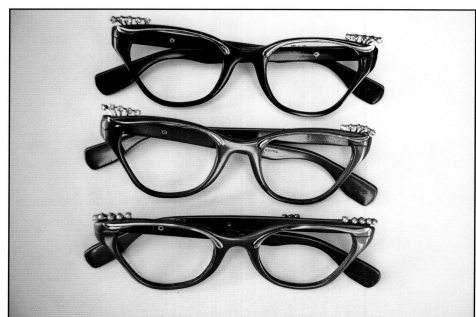

Top left: Tantalizing Turas in black with gold braid trim on brow. $140-160.

Top right: A gold-shaded Tura "Exclusive" with etched swirls on brow. $80-90.

Bottom left: Tura's "# 307" in bronze, with golden leaf on each brow. $100-115.

Bottom right: A Tura trio, each with decorative sprigs on brow edge. $100-115 each.

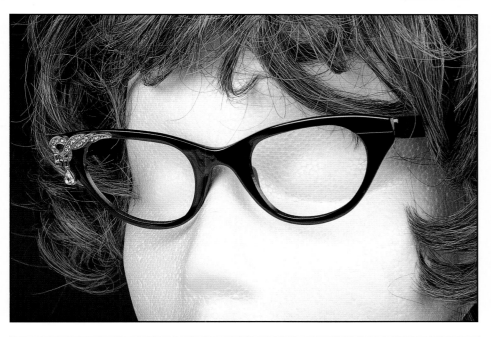

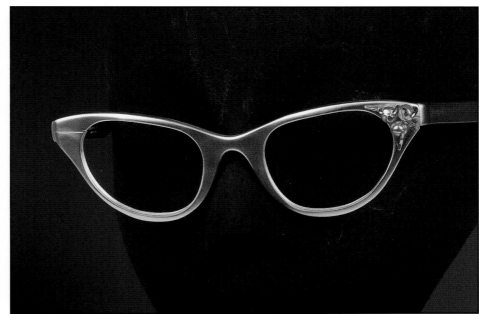

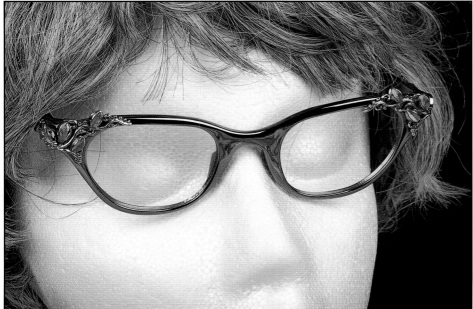

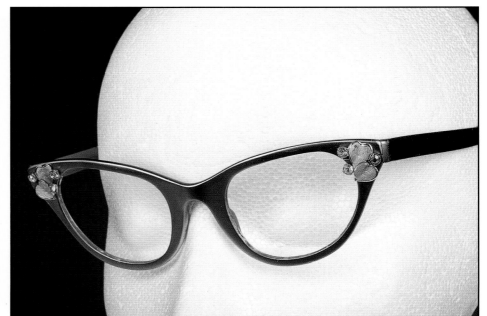

Top left: Rhinestone drops on right brow highlight a dark bronze Tura design. $150-170.

Top right: This time it's the left brow: Turas in silver pink, with three-pearl accent. $120-135.

Bottom left: Turas in bronze, with applied vines in gold and silver. $140-160.

Bottom right: Stunning steely-blue Tura pair, with hearts and rhinestone appliqué. $120-135.

More Tura hearts and rhinestones. $120-135.

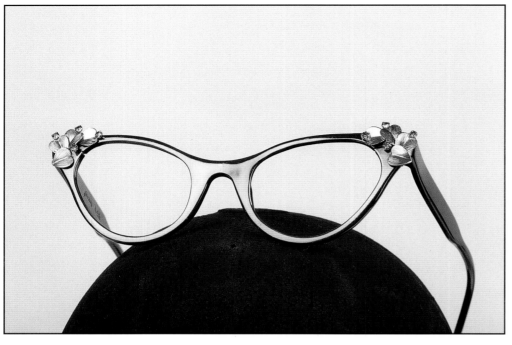

TRANS-WORLD Women's Zyl

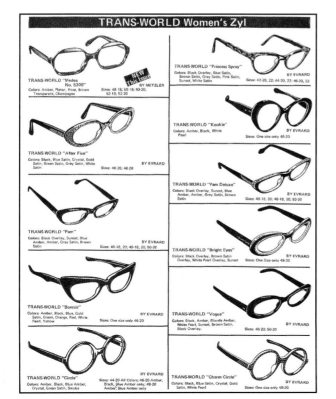

TRANS-WORLD "Medea No. 5300" NEW This Issue
Colors: Amber, Matar, Rose, Brown Transparent, Champagne
BY METZLER
Sizes: 48-18; 50-18; 50-20; 52-18; 52-20

TRANS-WORLD "After Five"
Colors: Black, Blue Satin, Crystal, Gold Satin, Green Satin, Grey Satin, White Satin
BY EVRARD
Sizes: 46-20; 48-20

TRANS-WORLD "Pam"
Colors: Black Overlay, Sunset, Blue Amber, Amber, Grey Satin, Brown Satin
BY EVRARD
Sizes: 46-18, 20; 48-18, 20; 50-20

TRANS-WORLD "Bonnie"
Colors: Amber, Black, Blue, Gold Satin, Green, Orange, Red, White Pearl, Yellow
BY EVRARD
Sizes: One size only 46-20

TRANS-WORLD "Circle"
Colors: Amber, Black, Blue Amber, Crystal, Green Satin, Smoke
BY EVRARD
Sizes: 44-20 All Colors; 46-20 Black, Blue Amber only; 48-20 Amber, Blue Amber only

TRANS-WORLD "Princess Spray"
Colors: Black Overlay, Blue Satin, Brown Satin, Grey Satin, Pink Satin, Sunset, White Satin
BY EVRARD
Sizes: 42-20, 22; 44-20, 22; 46-20, 22

TRANS-WORLD "Kookie"
Colors: Amber, Black, White Pearl
BY EVRARD
Sizes: One size only 46-20

TRANS-WORLD "Pam Deluxe"
Colors: Black Overlay, Sunset, Blue Amber, Amber, Grey Satin, Brown Satin
BY EVRARD
Sizes: 46-18, 20; 48-18, 20; 50-20

TRANS-WORLD "Bright Eyes"
Colors: Black Overlay, Brown Satin Overlay, White Pearl Overlay, Sunset
BY EVRARD
Sizes: One Size only 48-20

TRANS-WORLD "Vogue"
Colors: Black, Amber, Blonde Amber, White Pearl, Sunset, Brown Satin, Black Overlay
BY EVRARD
Sizes: 48-20; 50-20

TRANS-WORLD "Charm Circle"
Colors: Black, Amber, Crystal, Gold Satin, White Pearl
BY EVRARD
Sizes: One size only 48-20

TRANS-WORLD Women's Zyl

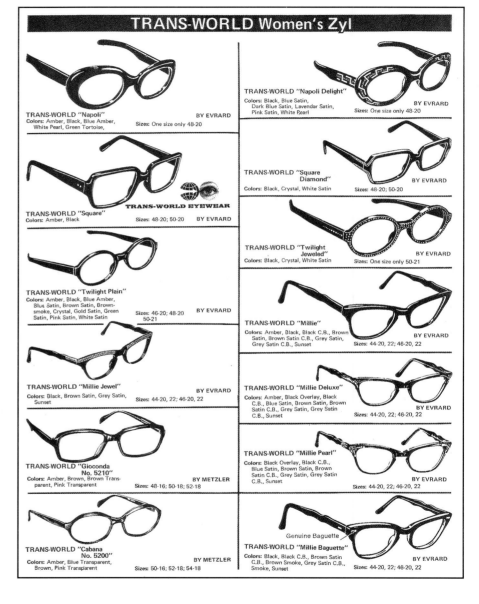

TRANS-WORLD "Napoli"
Colors: Amber, Black, Blue Amber, White Pearl, Green Tortoise,
BY EVRARD
Sizes: One size only 48-20

TRANS-WORLD "Square"
Colors: Amber, Black
BY EVRARD
Sizes: 48-20; 50-20

TRANS-WORLD EYEWEAR

TRANS-WORLD "Twilight Plain"
Colors: Amber, Black, Blue Amber, Blue Satin, Brown Satin, Brown-smoke, Crystal, Gold Satin, Green Satin, Pink Satin, White Satin
BY EVRARD
Sizes: 46-20; 48-20 50-21

TRANS-WORLD "Millie Jewel"
Colors: Black, Brown Satin, Grey Satin, Sunset
BY EVRARD
Sizes: 44-20, 22; 46-20, 22

TRANS-WORLD "Gioconda No. 5210"
Colors: Amber, Brown, Brown Transparent, Pink Transparent
BY METZLER
Sizes: 48-16; 50-18; 52-18

TRANS-WORLD "Cabana No. 5200"
Colors: Amber, Blue Transparent, Brown, Pink Transparent
BY METZLER
Sizes: 50-16; 52-18; 54-18

TRANS-WORLD "Napoli Delight"
Colors: Black, Blue Satin, Dark Blue Satin, Lavendar Satin, Pink Satin, White Pearl
BY EVRARD
Sizes: One size only 48-20

TRANS-WORLD "Square Diamond"
Colors: Black, Crystal, White Satin
BY EVRARD
Sizes: 48-20; 50-20

TRANS-WORLD "Twilight Jeweled"
Colors: Black, Crystal, White Satin
BY EVRARD
Sizes: One size only 50-21

TRANS-WORLD "Millie"
Colors: Amber, Black, Black C.B., Brown Satin, Brown Satin C.B., Grey Satin, Grey Satin C.B., Sunset
BY EVRARD
Sizes: 44-20, 22; 46-20, 22

TRANS-WORLD "Millie Deluxe"
Colors: Amber, Black Overlay, Black C.B., Blue Satin, Brown Satin, Brown Satin C.B., Grey Satin, Grey Satin C.B., Sunset
BY EVRARD
Sizes: 44-20, 22; 46-20, 22

TRANS-WORLD "Millie Pearl"
Colors: Black Overlay, Black C.B., Blue Satin, Brown Satin, Brown Satin C.B., Grey Satin, Grey Satin C.B., Sunset
BY EVRARD
Sizes: 44-20, 22; 46-20, 22

Genuine Baguette
TRANS-WORLD "Millie Baguette"
Colors: Black, Black C.B., Brown Satin C.B., Brown Smoke, Grey Satin C.B., Smoke, Sunset
BY EVRARD
Sizes: 44-20, 22; 46-20, 22

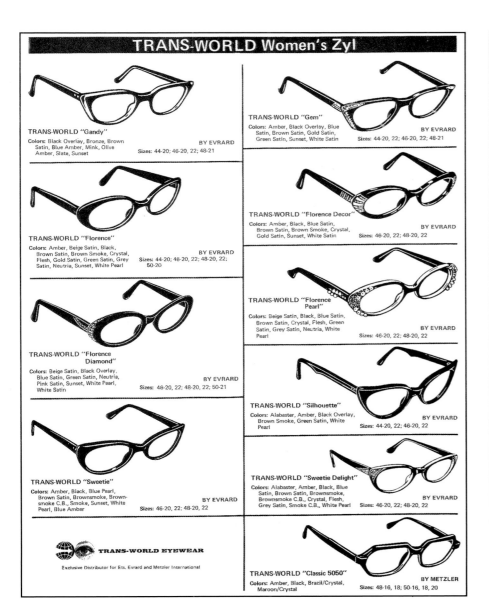

TRANS-WORLD "Gandy"

Colors: Black Overlay, Bronze, Brown Satin, Blue Amber, Mink, Olive Amber, Slate, Sunset

BY EVRARD

Sizes: 44-20; 46-20, 22; 48-21

TRANS-WORLD "Florence"

Colors: Amber, Beige Satin, Black, Brown Satin, Brown Smoke, Crystal, Flesh, Gold Satin, Green Satin, Grey Satin, Neutria, Sunset, White Pearl

BY EVRARD

Sizes: 44-20; 46-20, 22; 48-20, 22; 50-20

TRANS-WORLD "Florence Diamond"

Colors: Beige Satin, Black Overlay, Blue Satin, Green Satin, Neutria, Pink Satin, Sunset, White Pearl, White Satin

BY EVRARD

Sizes: 46-20, 22; 48-20, 22; 50-21

TRANS-WORLD "Sweetie"

Colors: Amber, Black, Blue Pearl, Brown Satin, Brownsmoke, Brown-smoke C.B., Smoke, Sunset, White Pearl, Blue Amber

BY EVRARD

Sizes: 46-20, 22; 48-20, 22

TRANS-WORLD EYEWEAR

Exclusive Distributor for Ets. Evrard and Metzler International

TRANS-WORLD "Gem"

Colors: Amber, Black Overlay, Blue Satin, Brown Satin, Gold Satin, Green Satin, Sunset, White Satin

BY EVRARD

Sizes: 44-20, 22; 46-20, 22; 48-21

TRANS-WORLD "Florence Decor"

Colors: Amber, Black, Blue Satin, Brown Satin, Brown Smoke, Crystal, Gold Satin, Sunset, White Satin

BY EVRARD

Sizes: 46-20, 22; 48-20, 22

TRANS-WORLD "Florence Pearl"

Colors: Beige Satin, Black, Blue Satin, Brown Satin, Crystal, Flesh, Green Satin, Grey Satin, Neutria, White Pearl

BY EVRARD

Sizes: 46-20, 22; 48-20, 22

TRANS-WORLD "Silhouette"

Colors: Alabaster, Amber, Black Overlay, Brown Smoke, Green Satin, White Pearl

BY EVRARD

Sizes: 44-20, 22; 46-20, 22

TRANS-WORLD "Sweetie Delight"

Colors: Alabaster, Amber, Black, Blue Satin, Brown Satin, Brownsmoke, Brownsmoke C.B., Crystal, Flesh, Grey Satin, Smoke C.B., White Pearl

BY EVRARD

Sizes: 46-20, 22; 48-20, 22

TRANS-WORLD "Classic 5050"

Colors: Amber, Black, Brazil/Crystal, Maroon/Crystal

BY METZLER

Sizes: 48-16, 18; 50-16, 18, 20

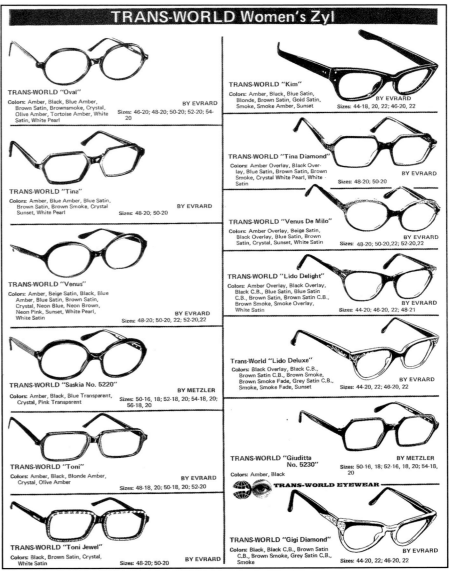

TRANS-WORLD "Oval"

Colors: Amber, Black, Blue Amber, Brown Satin, Brownsmoke, Crystal, Olive Amber, Tortoise Amber, White Satin, White Pearl

BY EVRARD

Sizes: 46-20; 48-20; 50-20; 52-20; 54-20

TRANS-WORLD "Tina"

Colors: Amber, Blue Amber, Blue Satin, Brown Satin, Brown Smoke, Crystal Sunset, White Pearl

BY EVRARD

Sizes: 48-20; 50-20

TRANS-WORLD "Venus"

Colors: Amber, Beige Satin, Black, Blue Amber, Blue Satin, Green Satin, Crystal, Neon Blue, Neon Brown, Neon Pink, Sunset, White Pearl, White Satin

BY EVRARD

Sizes: 48-20; 50-20, 22; 52-20, 22

TRANS-WORLD "Saskia No. 5220"

Colors: Amber, Black, Blue Transparent, Crystal, Pink Transparent

BY METZLER

Sizes: 50-16, 18; 52-18, 20; 54-18, 20; 56-18, 20

TRANS-WORLD "Toni"

Colors: Amber, Black, Blonde Amber, Crystal, Olive Amber

BY EVRARD

Sizes: 48-18, 20; 50-18, 20; 52-20

TRANS-WORLD "Toni Jewel"

Colors: Black, Brown Satin, Crystal, White Satin

BY EVRARD

Sizes: 48-20; 50-20

TRANS-WORLD "Kim"

Colors: Amber, Black, Blue Satin, Blonde, Brown Satin, Gold Satin, Smoke, Smoke Amber, Sunset

BY EVRARD

Sizes: 44-18, 20, 22; 46-20, 22

TRANS-WORLD "Tina Diamond"

Colors: Amber Overlay, Black Overlay, Blue Satin, Brown Satin, Brown Smoke, Crystal White Pearl, White Satin

BY EVRARD

Sizes: 48-20; 50-20

TRANS-WORLD "Venus De Milo"

Colors: Amber Overlay, Beige Satin, Black Overlay, Blue Satin, Brown Satin, Crystal, Sunset, White Satin

BY EVRARD

Sizes: 48-20; 50-20,22; 52-20,22

TRANS-WORLD "Lido Delight"

Colors: Amber Overlay, Black Overlay, Black C.B., Blue Satin, Blue Satin C.B., Brown Satin, Brown Satin C.B., Brown Smoke, Smoke Overlay, White Satin

BY EVRARD

Sizes: 44-20; 46-20, 22; 48-21

Trans-World "Lido Deluxe"

Colors: Black Overlay, Black C.B., Brown Satin C.B., Brown Smoke, Brown Smoke Fade, Grey Satin C.B., Smoke, Smoke Fade, Sunset

BY EVRARD

Sizes: 44-20, 22; 46-20, 22

TRANS-WORLD "Giuditta No. 5230"

Colors: Amber, Black

BY METZLER

Sizes: 50-16, 18; 52-16, 18, 20; 54-18, 20

TRANS-WORLD EYEWEAR

TRANS-WORLD "Gigi Diamond"

Colors: Black, Black C.B., Brown Satin C.B., Brown Smoke, Grey Satin C.B., Smoke

BY EVRARD

Sizes: 44-20, 22; 46-20, 22

This page and opposite: Style samplings by Trans-World Eyewear Corporation (TWEC/TWE), distributors for Evrard "Frame France" and Metzler.

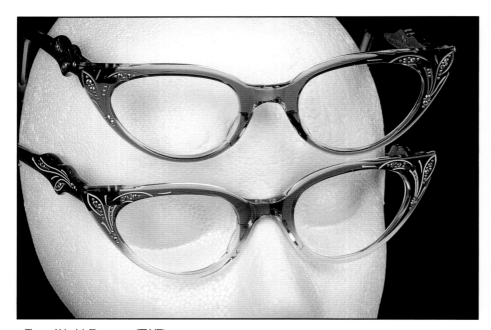

Trans-World Eyewear (TWE) "Cutie Spray" in gold and gray. $70-85 each.

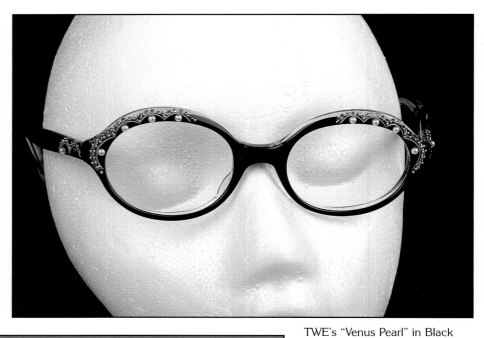

TWE's "Venus Pearl" in Black Overlay. $70-85.

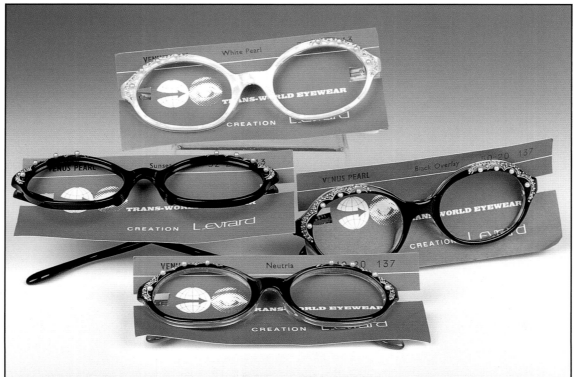

A "Venus Pearl" selection in White Pearl, Sunset, Black Overlay, and Neutria. $70-85 each

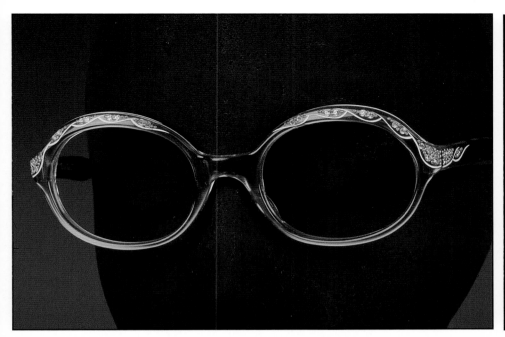

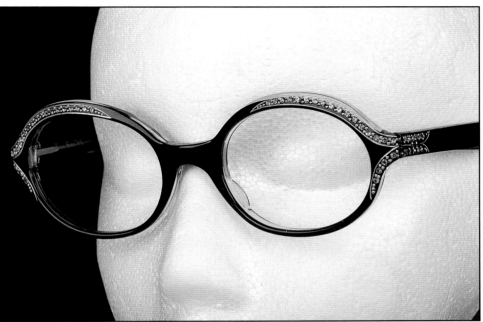

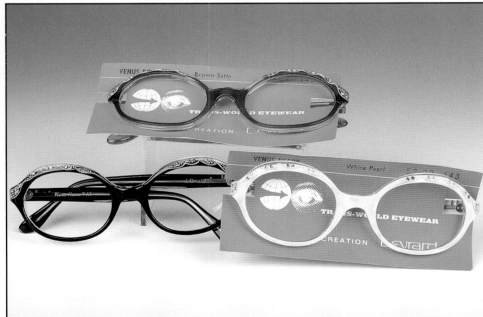

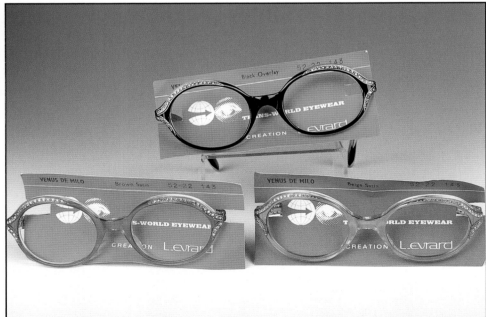

Top left: "Venus Decor" by TWE in Brown Satin. $70-85

Bottom left: Three "Venus Decor" choices: Brown Satin, Black Overlay, and White Pearl. $70-85 each.

Top right: More Venus: TWE's "Venus De Milo" in Black Overlay. $70-85.

Bottom right: A "Venus De Milo" assortment: Black Overlay, Brown Satin, Beige Satin. $70-85 each.

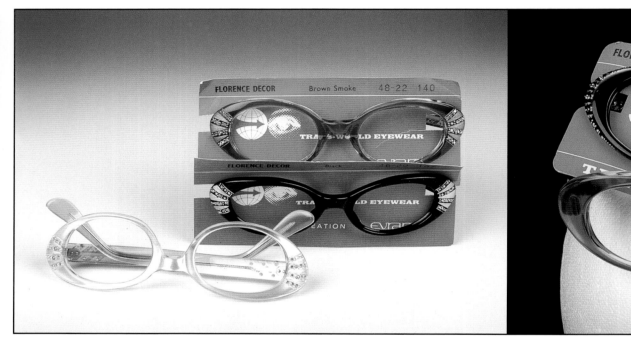

"Florence Decor" by TWE, shown here in Brown Smoke, Black, and White Pearl. $70-85 each.

TWE's "Florence Diamond" in Sunset and Blue Satin. $70-85 each.

Opposite page:
Left: Who thinks up these titles? TWE's "Sweetie Delight," shown (*from front*) in White Pearl, Black Overlay, Tortoise Overlay, and Smoke. $70-85 each.

Right: More sweet things: "Sweetie Delight" in Clear Pink, Light Blue, and Silver. $70-85 each.

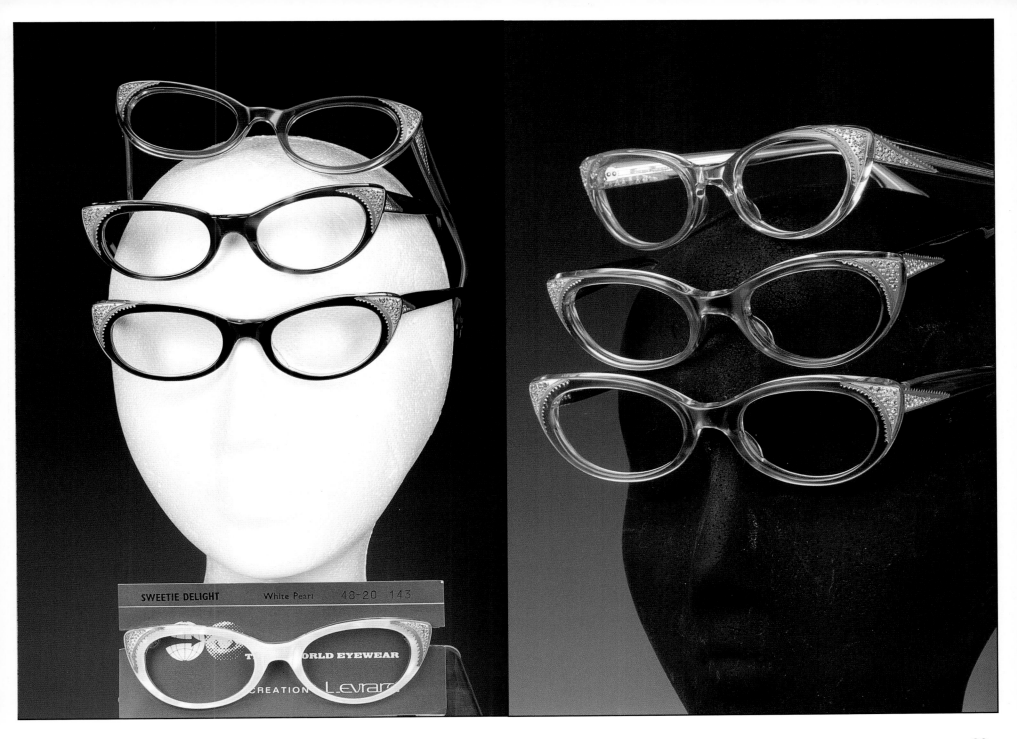

SWEETIE DELIGHT   White Pearl   48-20 143

WORLD EYEWEAR

CREATION Levrard

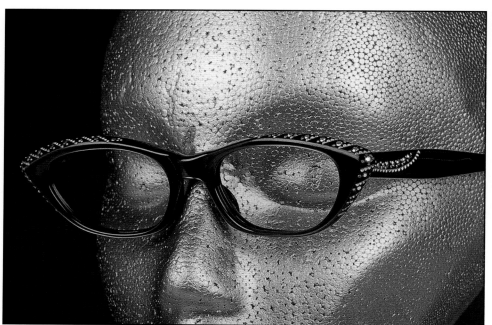

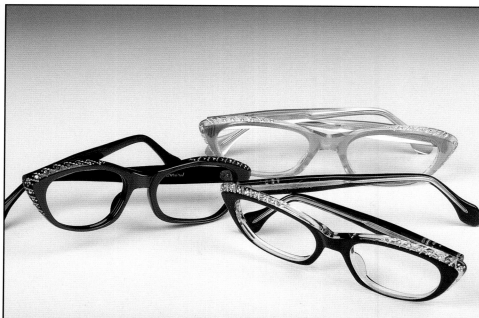

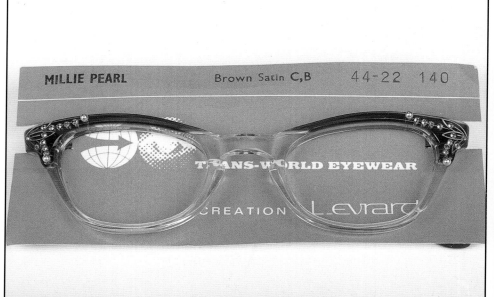

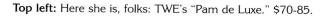

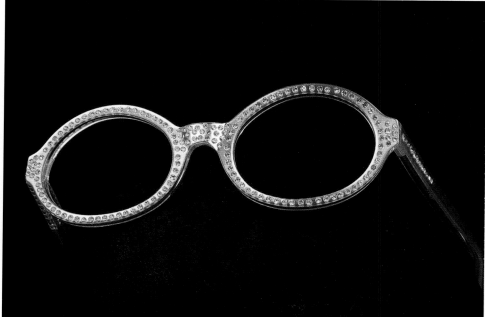

Top left: Here she is, folks: TWE's "Pam de Luxe." $70-85.

Top right: "Pam de Luxe" in Amber, Smoke, and Black Overlay. $70-85 each.

Bottom left: Can this be a play on words? TWE's "Millie Pearl" (not "Minnie") by Evrard, in Brown Satin. $70-85.

Bottom right: Sure to sparkle: "Twilight Jewel" by TWE, in White Pearl. $70-85.

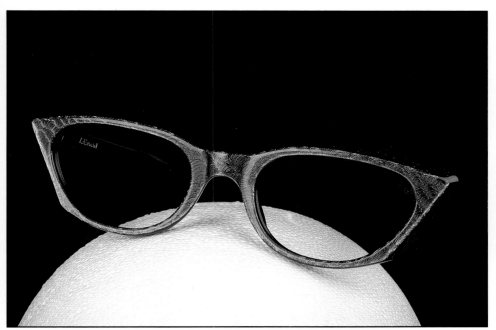

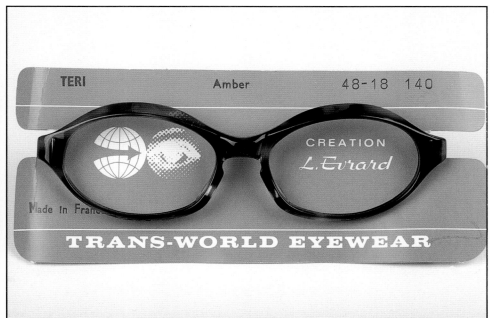

Top left: Good enough to eat: TWE's "Candy" in Bronze. $70-85.

Top right: "Teri" by TWE, in amber. $70-85.

Bottom: Also "Teri," but in Tortoise Amber. $70-85.

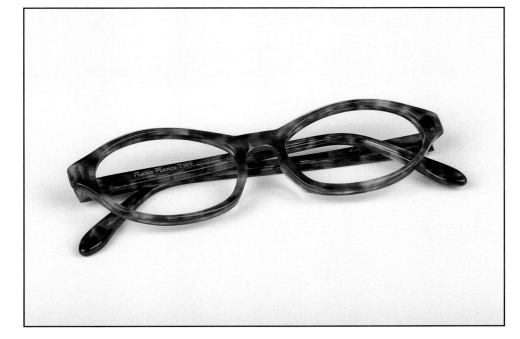

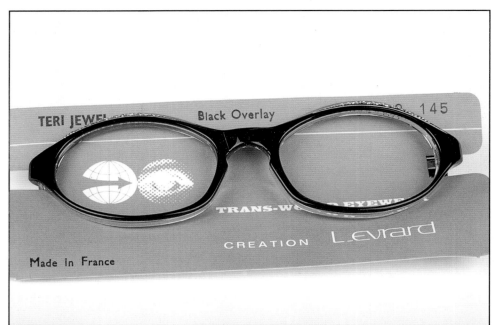

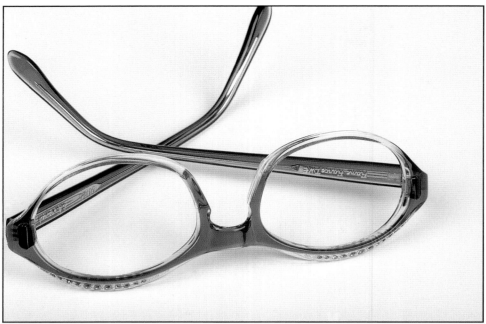

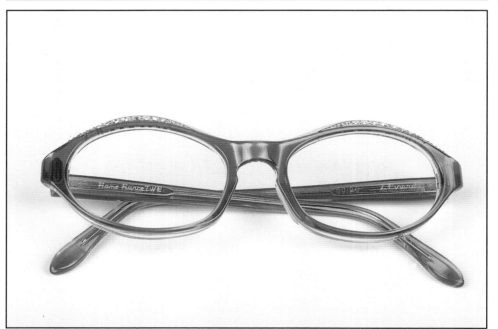

Top left: "Teri's" more decorative relative, "Teri Jewel," in Black Overlay. $70-85.

Top right: "Teri Jewel" in Smoke. $70-85

Bottom: More jewelry: "Teri Jewel" in Sunset. $70-85.

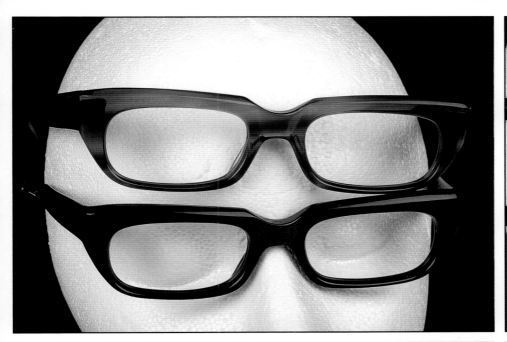

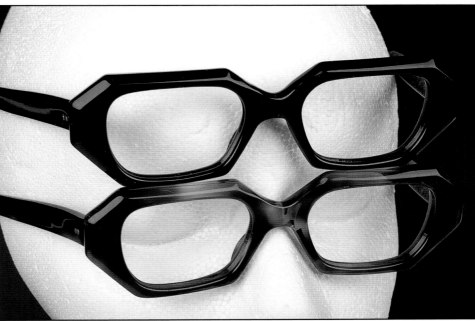

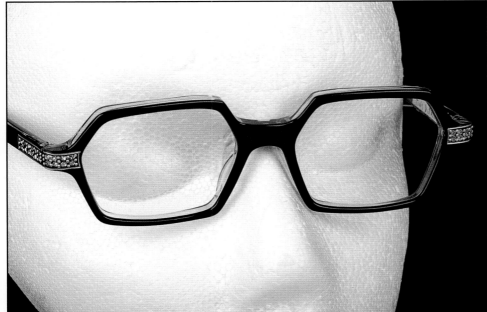

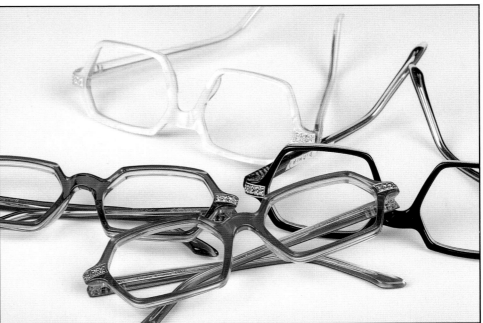

Top left: Just right for the office: TWE's "Secretary," in Black and Tortoise. $70-85 each.

Top right: At least the name has a South American flavor: TWE's "Brazil" in Black and Tortoise. $70-85 each.

Bottom left: For dressier occasions: "Tina Diamond" by TWE in Black Overlay. $70-85.

Bottom right: A "Tina Diamond" assortment: Smoke, Sunset, White Pearl, and Black Overlay. $70-85 each.

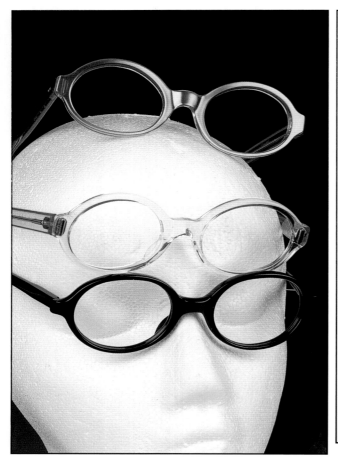

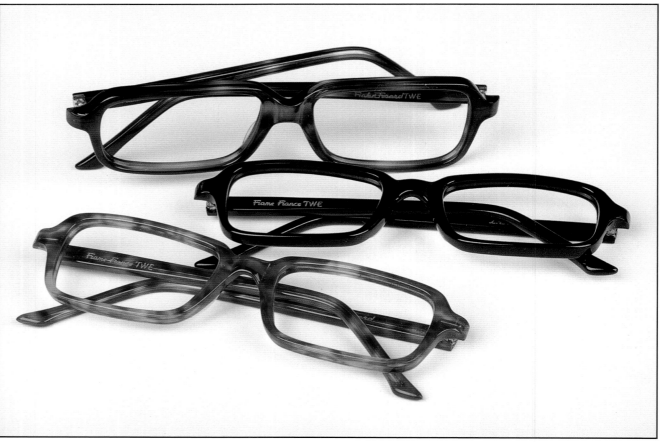

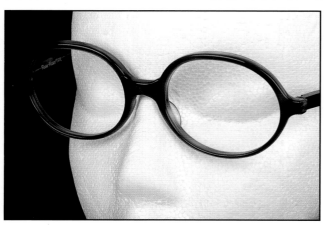

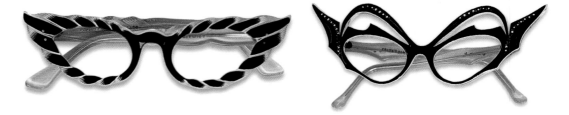

Top left: The title is self-explanatory: the TWE "Oval" in Light Blue, Clear, and Black. $70-85 each.

Bottom left: Another "Oval" in Tortoise. $70-85.

Top right: Say hello to "Toni," from TWE in Dark Amber, Black, and Blonde Amber. $70-85 each.

Bottom center: A unique TWE "Twist" cat-eye pair in black and clear. $90-100.

Bottom right: Another TWE Frame France curiosity: black cat-eye "highbrows" with rhinestone trim. $130-150.

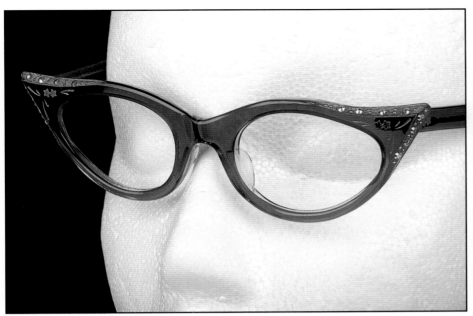

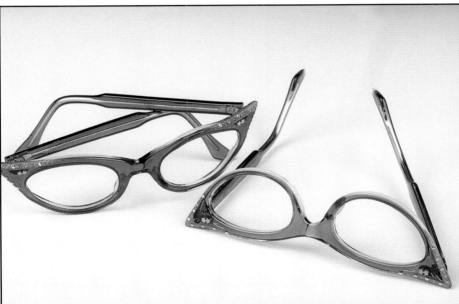

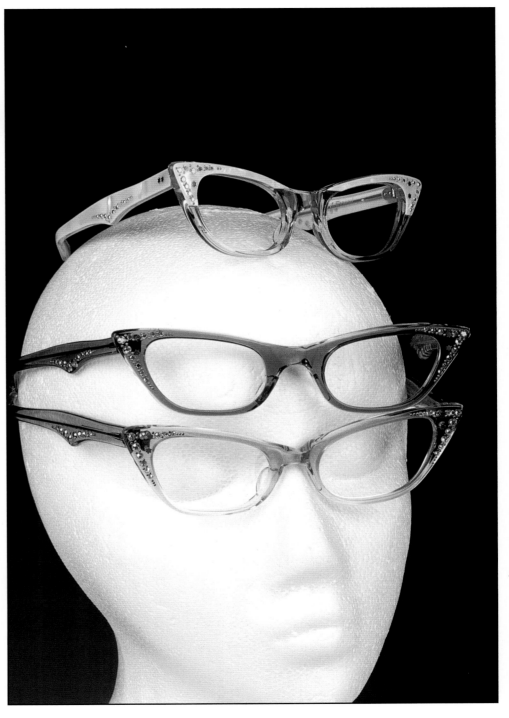

Top left: Rhinestones and gold trim accent a Victory cat-eye pair in Smoke. Star-shaped screw heads at the temple hinge are Victory hallmarks. $70-85.

Bottom left: The cat came back: Victory Smoke cat-eye joined by a pair in Light Blue. $70-85 each.

Right: V for Victory: dainty sprinkles of rhinestones adorn this Victory design in White Pearl, Sunset, and Blue. $70-85 each.

Eyeing the Small Fry

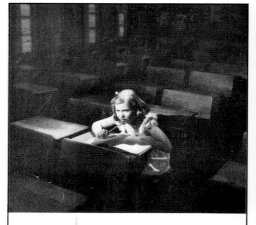

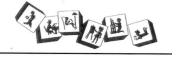

LITTLE LADY IN THE DARK

Young eyes groping in a fog . . . weary, worried eyes peering vainly at the blurred blackboard, straining over books that are always fuzzy . . . helpless, tear-filled eyes!

Unhappy little lady, trying so hard to learn and make Mummy and Daddy proud of her . . . so bewildered and ashamed at having to stay after school again!

Mother — or Dad — you must come to her rescue. There can be no greater handicap to your child than imperfect eyesight. Reliable help is readily available—and worth every cent it costs. To take your little lady — or little man — out of the dark and into the light of unclouded, flawless vision is such a simple thing.

Have the youngster's eyesight thoroughly examined by a qualified specialist who will prescribe scientific glasses, exercises or other visual aid, if necessary. Your child's vision is too precious to gamble with . . . so don't take a chance on "quickie," substandard eye-care. Those eyes deserve the best that ophthalmic science, technical skill and flawless materials can provide.

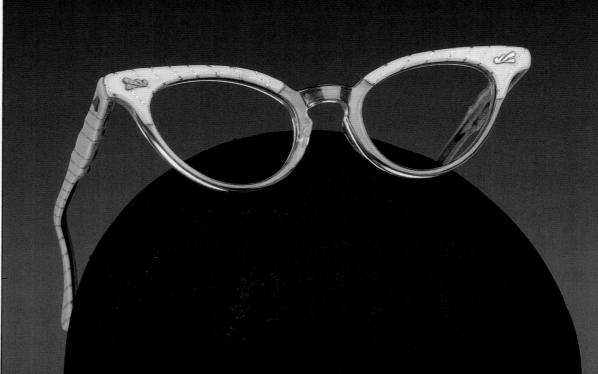

What girl wouldn't give her baby teeth for this pink plastic with gold-striped laminate by Graceline? $30-40.

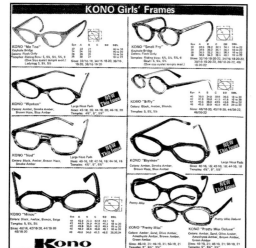

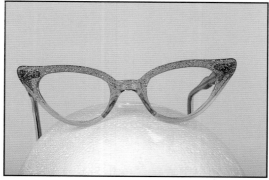

Top left: "Young eyes groping in a fog...weary worried eyes peering vainly at the blurred blackboard...helpless tear-filled eyes." Bausch & Lomb came on strong in 1953, encouraging parents to have their "little lady in the dark" tested for "imperfect eyesight." The 1950s saw a burgeoning market in children's eyewear, with manufacturers ready and willing to take squinting kiddies "out of the dark and into the light of unclouded, flawless vision."

Bottom left: Children's eyeglass styles often mimicked adult ones. Shown are several offered by Kono, circa 1972.

Bottom center: An unidentified manufacturer's gold glitter frame, guaranteed to set the boy-next-door's heart thumping. $30-40.

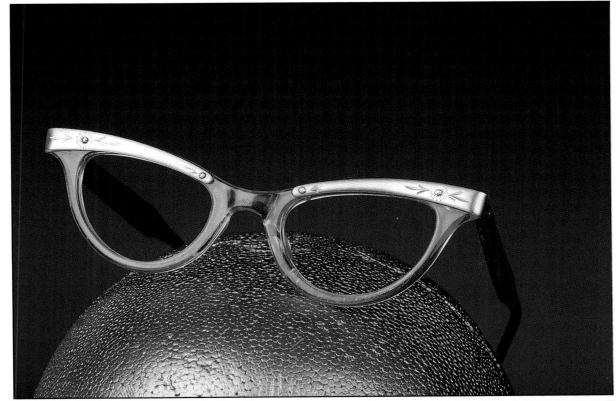

She's the envy of the playground in "Miss Terry Red," a pink and red stunner by Victory. $30-40.

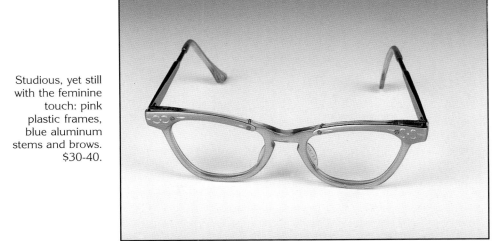

Studious, yet still with the feminine touch: pink plastic frames, blue aluminum stems and brows. $30-40.

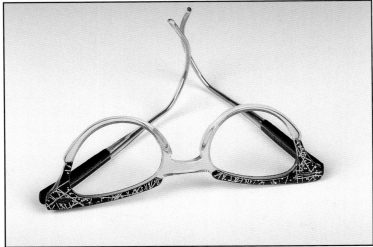

Something for the less shy: bold black glitter laminates by Bausch & Lomb. $30-40.

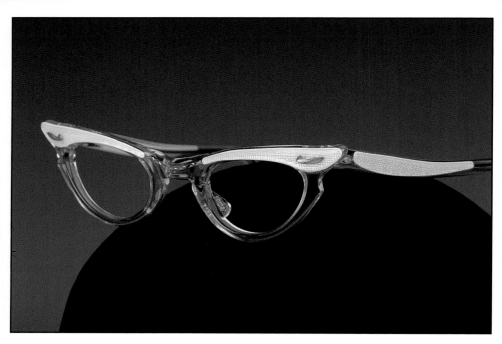

A sure thing from Shuron: clear plastic with white laminate brow and stem accents. $30-40.

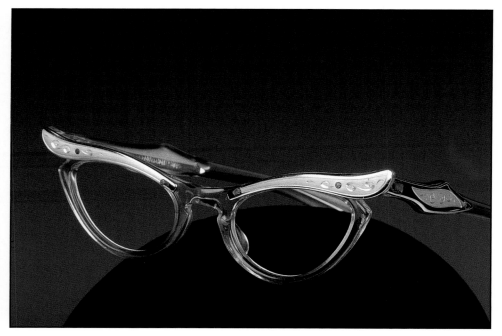

The Shuron idea from Marine, in clear plastic with applied aluminum brow and stem decor. $30-40.

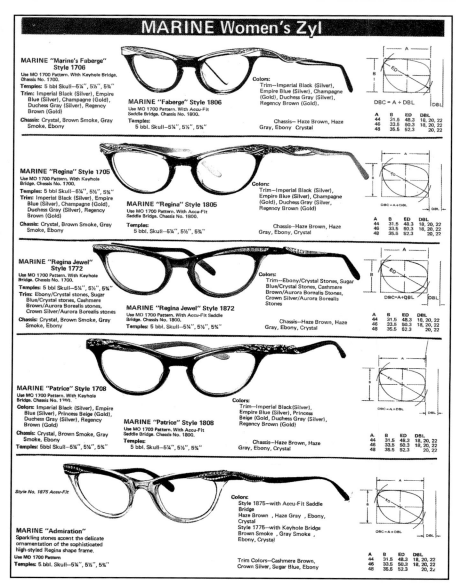

Like mother, like daughter: Marine's adult styles were echoed in its children's line.

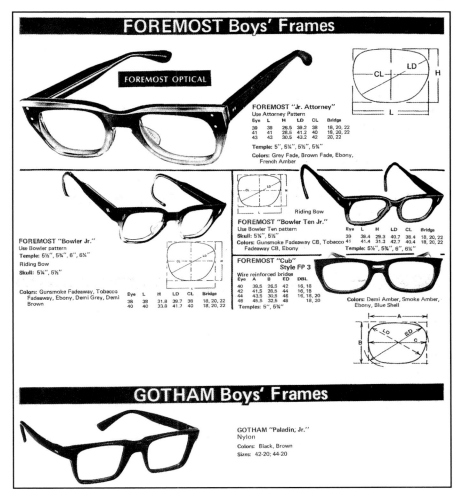

FOREMOST Boys' Frames

FOREMOST OPTICAL

FOREMOST "Jr. Attorney"
Use Attorney Pattern

Eye	L	H	LD	CL	Bridge
39	39	26.5	39.2	38	18, 20, 22
41	41	28.5	41.2	40	18, 20, 22
43	43	30.5	43.2	42	20, 22

Temple: 5", 5¼", 5½", 5¾"

Colors: Grey Fade, Brown Fade, Ebony, French Amber

Riding Bow

FOREMOST "Bowler Ten Jr."
Use Bowler Ten pattern
Skull: 5¼", 5½"
Colors: Gunsmoke Fadeaway CB, Tobacco Fadeaway CB, Ebony

Eye	L	H	LD	CL	Bridge
39	39.4	29.3	40.7	38.4	18, 20, 22
41	41.4	31.3	42.7	40.4	18, 20, 22

Temple: 5½", 5¾", 6", 6¼"

FOREMOST "Cub"
Style FP 3
Wire reinforced bridge

Eye	A	B	ED	DBL
40	39.5	26.5	42	16, 18
42	41.5	28.5	44	16, 18
44	43.5	30.5	46	16, 18, 20
46	46.5	32.5	48	18, 20

Temples: 5", 5¾"

Colors: Demi Amber, Smoke Amber, Ebony, Blue Shell

FOREMOST "Bowler Jr."
Use Bowler pattern
Temple: 5½", 5¾", 6", 6¼"
Riding Bow
Skull: 5¼", 5½"

Colors: Gunsmoke Fadeaway, Tobacco Fadeaway, Ebony, Demi Grey, Demi Brown

Eye	L	H	LD	CL	Bridge
38	38	31.8	39.7	38	18, 20, 22
40	40	33.8	41.7	40	18, 20, 22

GOTHAM Boys' Frames

GOTHAM "Paladin, Jr."
Nylon
Colors: Black, Brown
Sizes: 42-20; 44-20

BAUSCH & LOMB Men's

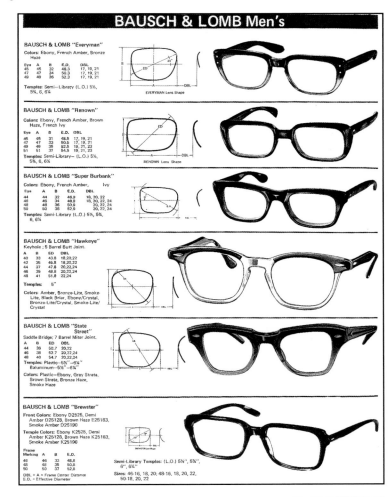

BAUSCH & LOMB "Everyman"
Colors: Ebony, French Amber, Bronze Haze

Eye	A	B	E.D.	DBL
45	45	32	48.3	17, 19, 21
47	47	34	50.3	17, 19, 21
49	49	36	52.3	17, 19, 21

Temples: Semi—Library (L.O.) 5½, 5¾, 6, 6¼
EVERYMAN Lens Shape

BAUSCH & LOMB "Renown"
Colors: Ebony, French Amber, Brown Haze, French Ivy

Eye	A	B	E.D.	DBL
45	45	31	48.5	17, 19, 21
47	47	33	50.5	17, 19, 21
49	49	35	52.5	19, 21, 23
51	51	37	54.5	19, 21, 23

Temples: Semi-Library— (L.O.) 5½, 5¾, 6, 6¼
RENOWN Lens Shape

BAUSCH & LOMB "Super Burbank"
Colors: Ebony, French Amber, Ivy

Eye	A	B	E.D.	DBL
44	44	32	46.9	18, 20, 22
46	46	34	48.9	18, 20, 22, 24
48	48	36	50.9	20, 22, 24
50	50	38	52.9	20, 22, 24

Temples: Semi-Library (L.O.) 5½, 5¾, 6, 6¼

BAUSCH & LOMB "Hawkeye"
Keyhole ; 5 Barrel Butt Joint.

A	B	ED	DBL
40	33	43.8	18,20,22
42	35	45.8	18,20,22
44	37	47.8	20,22,24
46	39	48.8	20,22,24
48	41	51.8	22,24

Temples: 5"
Colors: Amber, Bronze-Lite, Smoke-Lite, Black Briar, Ebony/Crystal, Bronze-Lite/Crystal, Smoke-Lite/Crystal

BAUSCH & LOMB "State Street"
Saddle Bridge; 7 Barrel Miter Joint.

A	B	ED	DBL
44	36	50.7	20,22
46	38	52.7	20,22,24
48	40	54.7	20,22,24

Temples: Plastic—5½"—6¼"
Baluminum—5½"—6¼"
Colors: Plastic—Ebony, Gray Strata, Brown Strata, Bronze Haze, Smoke Haze

BAUSCH & LOMB "Brewster"
Front Colors: Ebony D2525, Demi Amber D2512B, Brown Haze K25183, Smoke Amber D25190
Temple Colors: Ebony K2525, Demi Amber K2512B, Brown Haze K25183, Smoke Amber K25190

Frame Marking

	A	B	E.D.
46	46	33	48.8
48	48	35	50.8
50	50	37	52.8

Semi-Library Temples: (L.O.) 5½", 5¾", 6", 6¼"
Sizes: 46-16, 18, 20; 48-16, 18, 20, 22, 50-18, 20, 22

DBL + A = Frame Center Distance
E.D. = Effective Diameter

Above: Boys had fewer eyewear styles to choose from, though rugged-sounding model names did their best to compensate. Foremost offered "Jr. Attorney," "Bowler Jr.," and "Cub," while Gotham embraced the wild and wooly West with the heroic "Paladin, Jr."

Left: Grown-up boys fared slightly better. Shown is that rarity from the mid-'50s: a Bausch & Lomb ad including a male model! The B & L "Balrim" was available in both men's and women's versions.

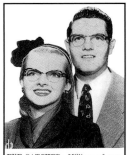

EYE-CATCHER: Millions of people have seen this beautiful color ad and display placard that heralds the Balrim and Balrim Citation.

Above: More of those hearty-sounding glasses for the guys: "Everyman," "Renown," "Super Burbank," "Hawkeye," and...well, you get the picture.

Right: Fortunately, B & L had a walking advertisement for its men's line in the form of popular television entertainer Steve Allen. In addition to crowning "Miss Specs" for several years, Mr. Allen also, according to the *Balco News*, wore "specs made up by B & L's New York prescription lab."

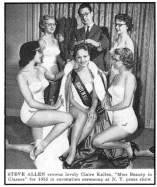

STEVE ALLEN crowns lovely Claire Kallen, "Miss Beauty in Glasses" for 1955 in coronation ceremony at N. Y. press show.

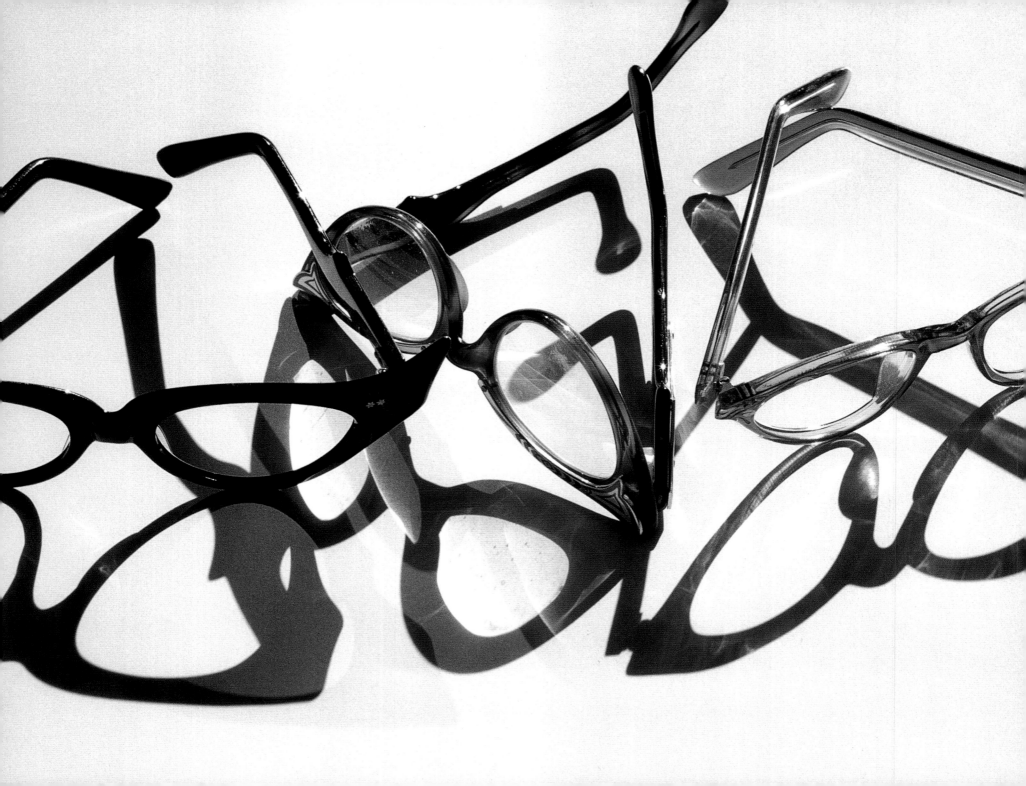

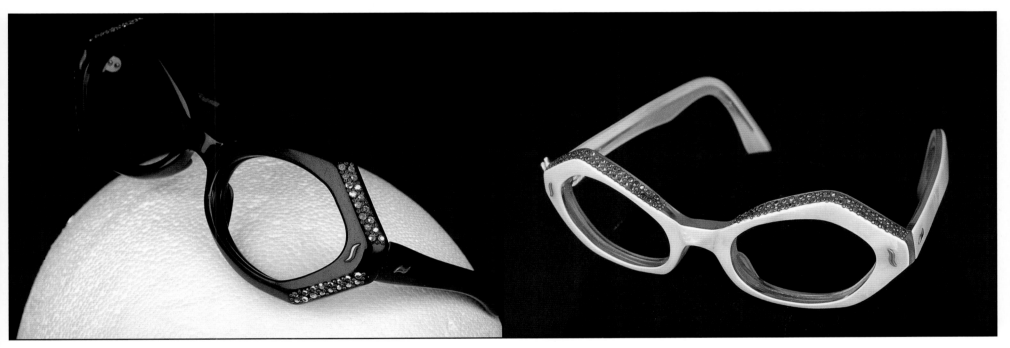

An arresting French design in black, with irregular-shaped frames, and rhinestone trim. $45-55.

The same in white. $45-55.

Opposite page: Some of the most exciting eyewear designs of the 1950s and '60s came from overseas. Shown, a simply styled French assortment. $50-75 each.

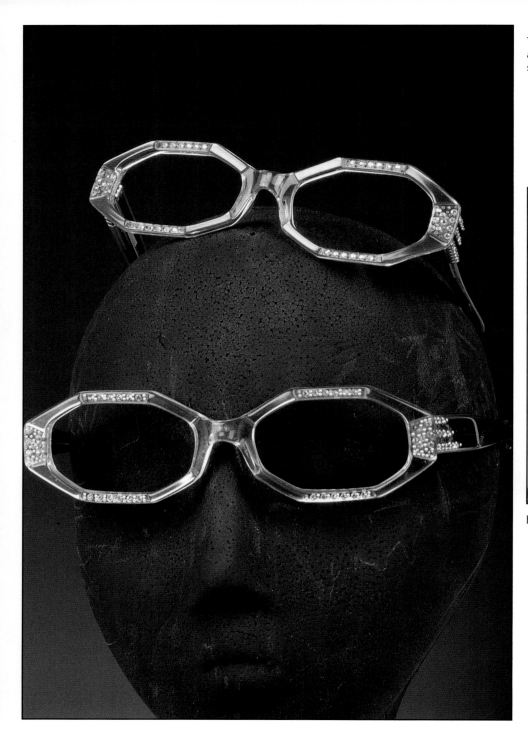

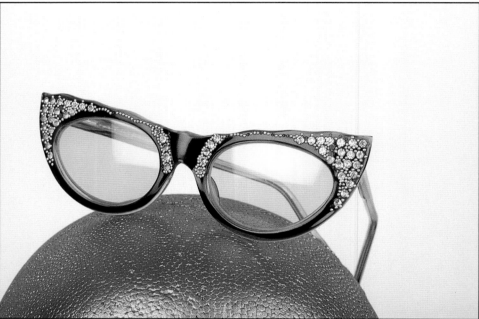

The French eye for shapes: light blue and smokey octagons, with rhinestone ornamentation. $45-55 each.

French tortoise-shells, garnished with rhinestones and tiny silver balls. $90-110.

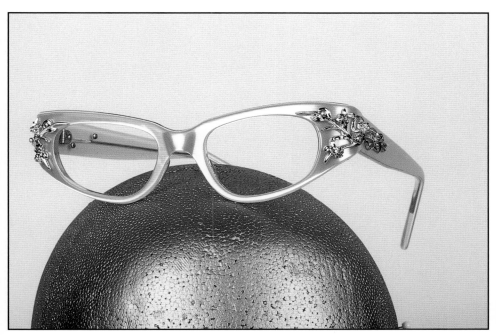

Yellow-gold pearlized plastic with gold floral appliqué—another French import. $120-135.

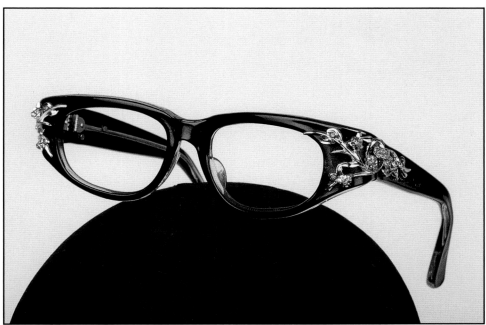

The same, this time in silver on black. $120-135.

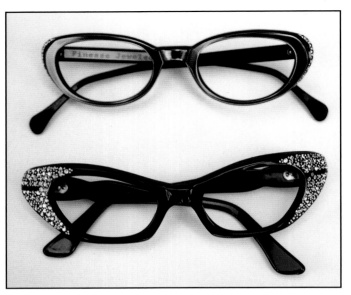

Just the thing for an evening at Moulin Rouge (or Las Vegas!) *Top:* frames in an unusual lavender shade. *Bottom:* frames heavily encrusted with rhinestones. $120-135 each.

Another "Hallmark," this time in sculptured pink. $120-130.

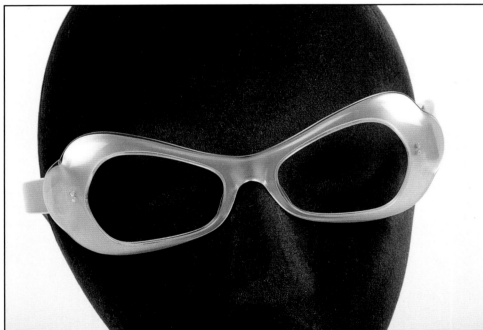

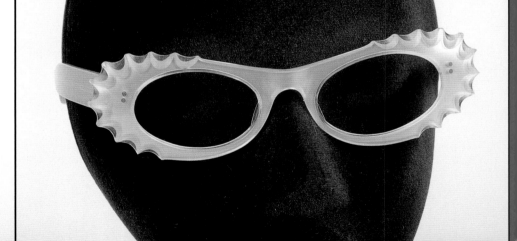

From 1955, blue sculptured "Hallmark," France. $120-130.

Another country heard from: the center bow tie-style frame hails from 1960s England. The top pair, with wood grain lamination, and the bottom, with multi-laminates, were made in France during the same period. Vive le différence! $100-120 each.

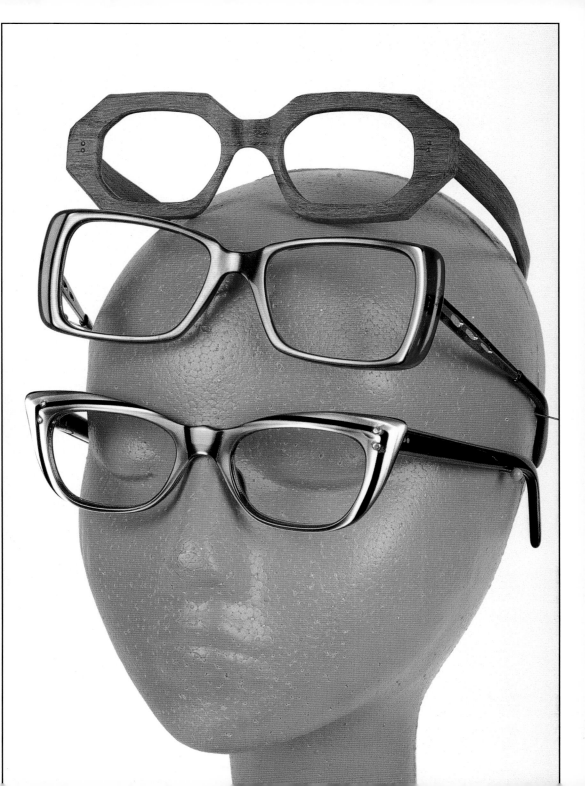

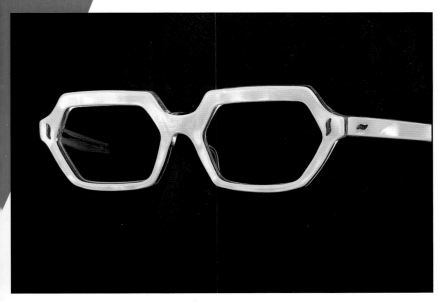

French hexagons, in white pearl. $45-55.

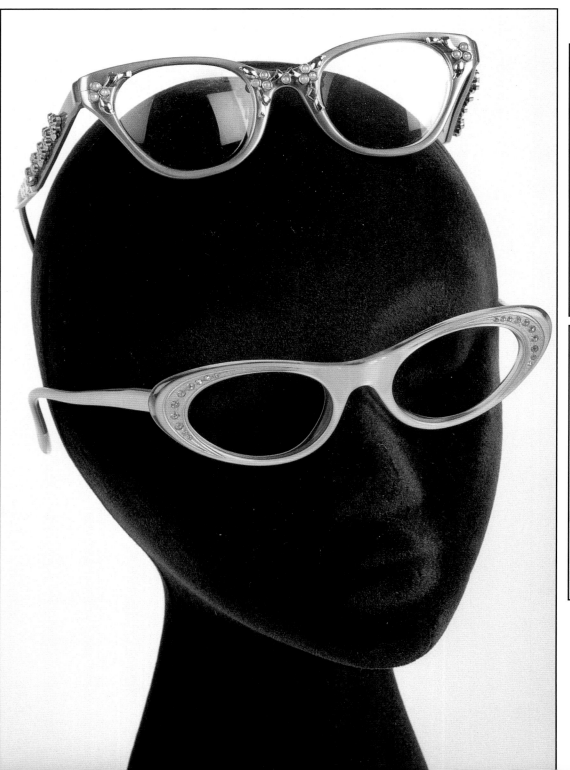

Designed to Please

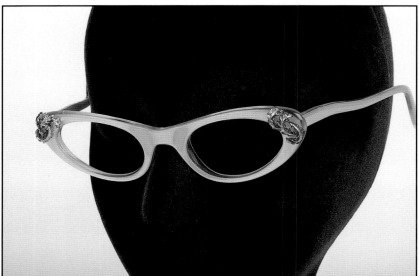

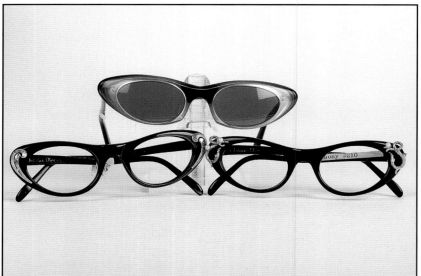

Top right: Over the years, name designers often turned to eyewear fashions, creating their own signature styles. These are by Christian Dior, $120-130.

Bottom right: The top pair are by TWE Frame France, the bottom two, in black with gold and jeweled ornament, are by Christian Dior. Top: $70-80. Bottom: $120-140 each.

Left: Tura, Tura, Tura! The ornately pearled Tura frames at top join a Christian Dior blonde pair, with light blue and rhinestone accents, at bottom. $80-100 each.

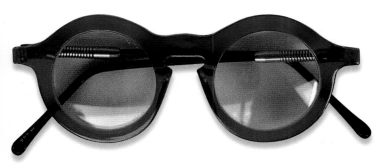

Courtesy of Hollywood's own Miss Edith Head. "High Tek Jr." in red. $225-250.

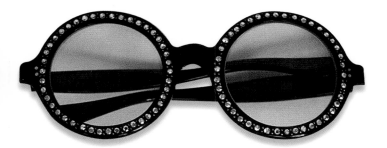

Oversize round black frames dotted with rhinestones, by Oleg Cassini. $100-125.

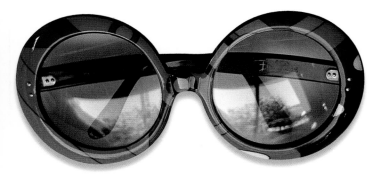

They're round—they're striped—they're spotted—they're a print pair by Emilio Pucci. $300-350.

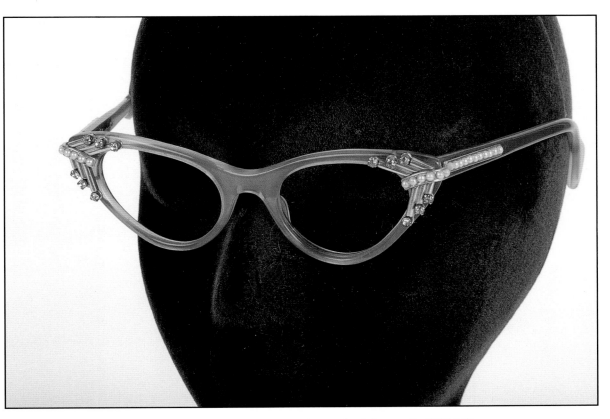

Elegantly pearled and rhinestoned frames by Schiaparelli. $230-250.

Pleasing To The Eye

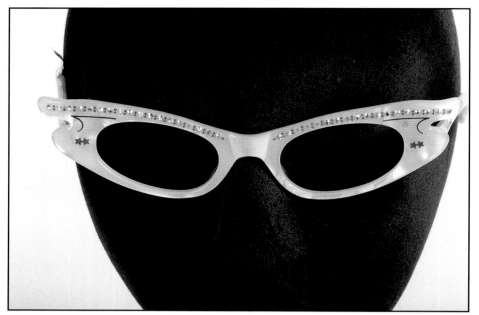

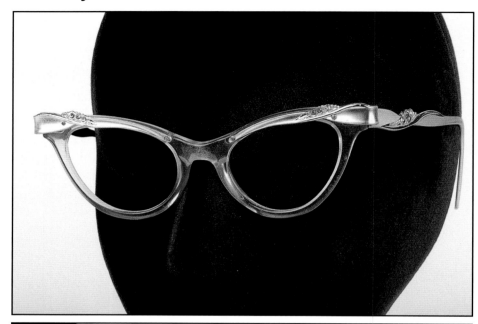

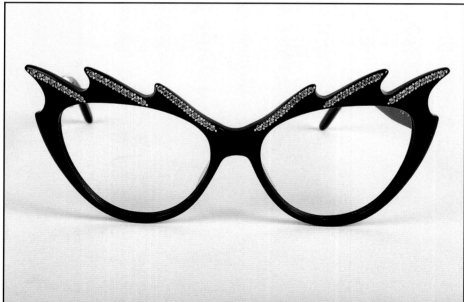

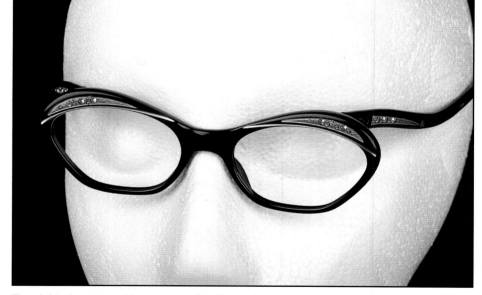

Top left: Some of the most intriguing designs defy classification. White pearlized "Jason" frames, with rhinestone brow. $90-100.

Bottom left: These Sortori Kaiia frames feature a zigzag brow with rhinestone ornament. $220-240.

Top right: A twisting rhinestone-studded brow design is carried through on the aluminum temples. The pair dates from the late 1950s. $100-125.

Bottom right: The unusual shape of these black-and-gold frames is augmented by temples attached to the interior of the brow, rather than at the brow edge. $70-80.

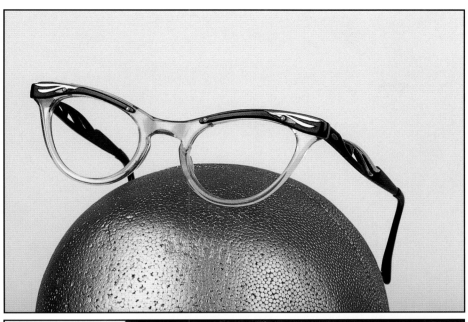

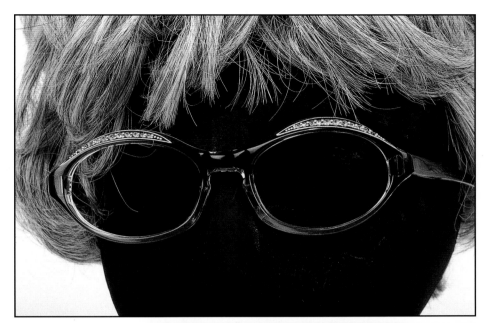

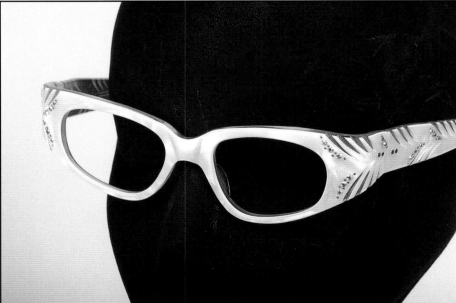

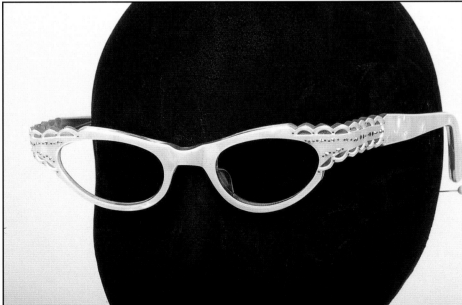

Top left: Another alluring combination frame, clear plastic with black aluminum brows and temples, and temple cutouts. $50-60.

Bottom left: Modified white cat-eyes, with cutaway slices at brow edge and temples. $90-110.

Top right: Smokey irregular ovals with rhinestone brows. $70-85.

Bottom right: White pearl, with rhinestone flourish and scalloped temples. $90-110.

59

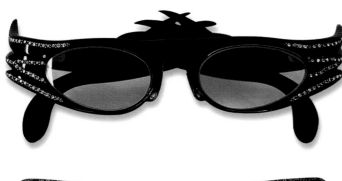

Black frames, with rhinestone corner curls, in the "Dame Edna" style. $80-90.

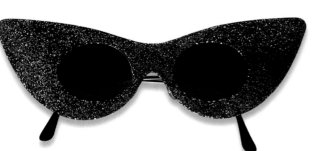

So Hollywood! The applied frame front is covered with purple iridescent glitter. $80-100.

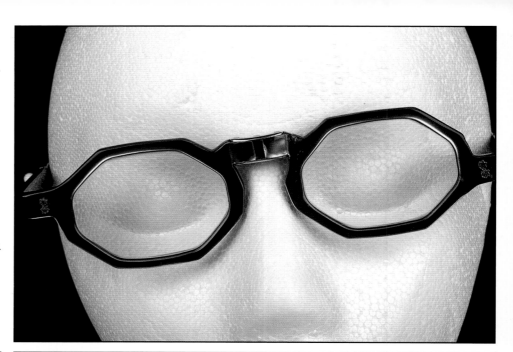

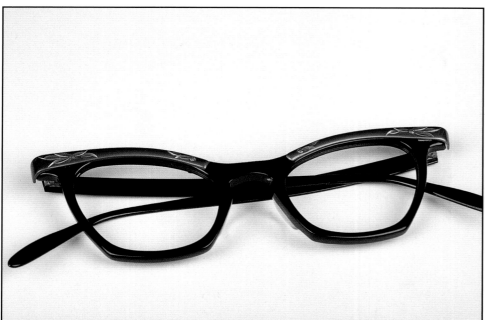

Black combinations, with green brow piece, gold and red leaf design. $50-60

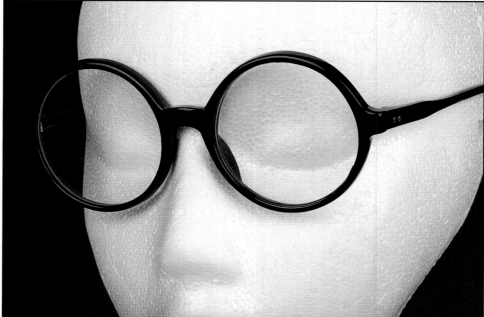

Top: A bit off the beaten path: silver octagons, $70-85.

Bottom: Wear them for a look of permanent surprise (or if you're George Burns): oversize circular frames, $70-85.

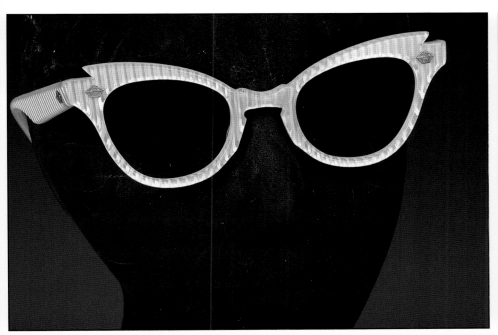

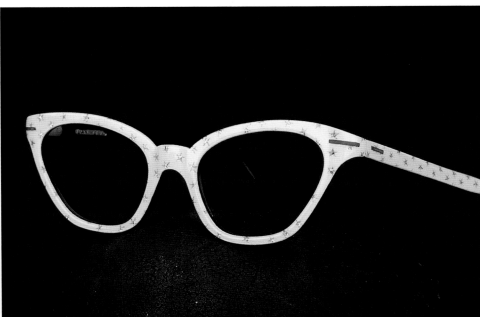

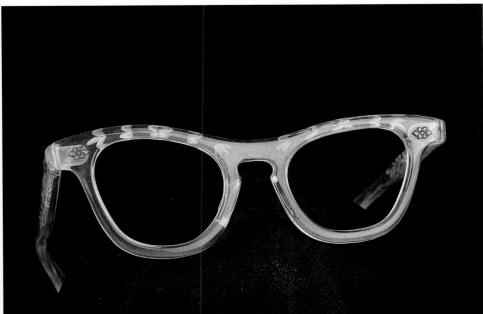

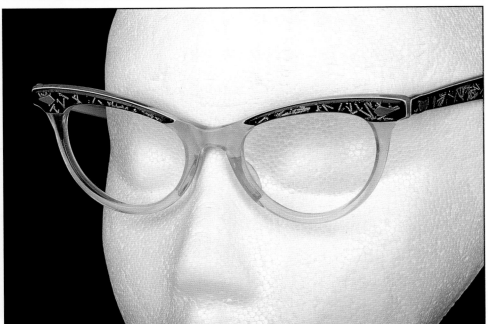

Top left: Made for summertime fun: pink stripes by Lumar. $90-105.

Bottom left: The frames and temples are clear; the design is carved on the reverse side. $75-85.

Top right: Are the stars out tonight? From Italy, by Lan-Cra, gold stars on white. $75-85.

Bottom right: Clear plastic with glitter bars on black brows and temples. $50-60.

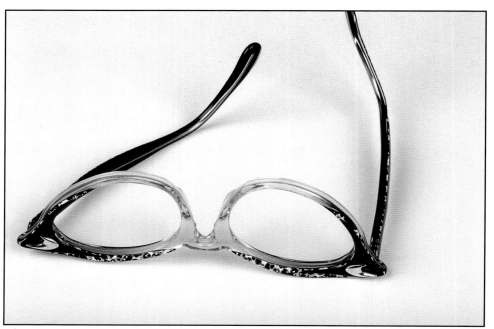

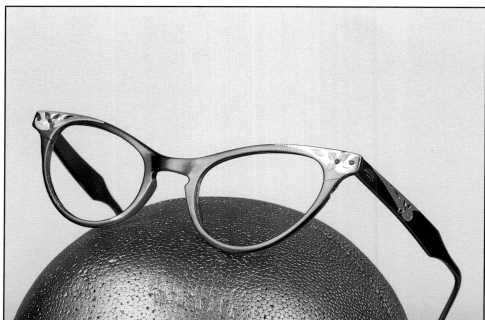

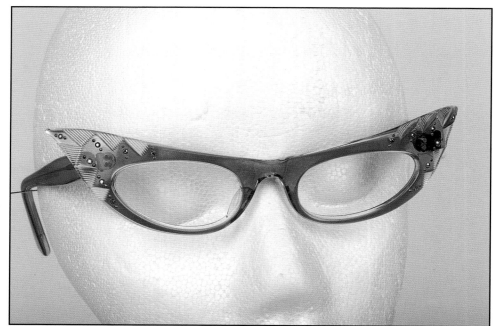

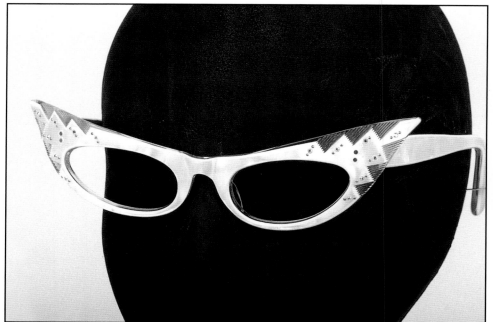

Top left: Beam me up! Clear plastic frames with black-and-white brow and temple pattern, crescent moon decorations at brow edge. $65-75.

Bottom left: Maybe not right for the office: a '50s icon, extreme cat-eyes, shown here in light blue, with clear cutaways and rhinestone trim. $70-80.

Top right: Now *this* is what the boss had in mind: decorous brown plastic frames, with just a hint of decoration at the brow edge and temples. $40-50.

Bottom right: On the other hand, cat-eyes can be so tempting, especially in pearlized white with clear cutaways and rhinestone trim. What's a girl to do? $70-80.

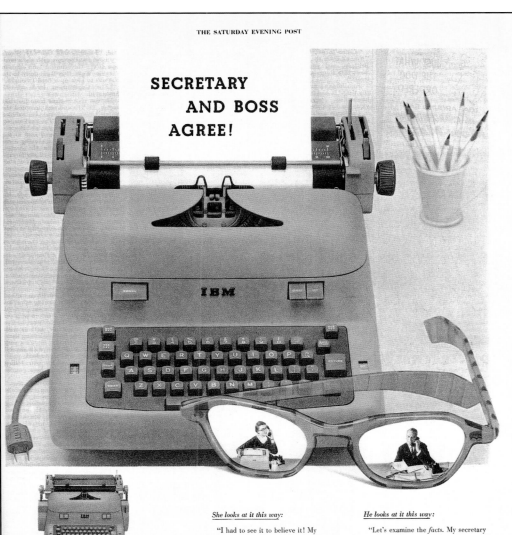

SECRETARY
AND BOSS
AGREE!

IBM

ONLY IBM MAKES A COMPLETE LINE
OF ELECTRIC TYPEWRITERS

This IBM EXECUTIVE Electric and the STANDARD Electric
shown above are just 2 of the 32 IBM models. They are available in many varied type faces and 7 handsome colors. Be sure
to see this exclusive IBM EXECUTIVE Electric—it makes your
letters look as if they were printed. For more information, call
your nearest IBM office or write IBM, 590 Madison Ave., New
York 22, N. Y. You're sure to go electric, make sure you go IBM!

She looks at it this way:

"I had to see it to believe it! My
new IBM Electric has made such a
change in my job . . . and in me! Now
I know what the IBM man meant
when he said that the IBM requires
95.4% less energy to operate than
my old manual typewriter. My work
goes so much faster—and it's
so much easier for me. There's no
'late-afternoon letdown' any more—
thanks to IBM 'power-typing'!"

He looks at it this way:

"Let's examine the *facts*. My secretary
has increased her work output over
15%—with less time and effort on
her part. So we've been able to handle
over 15% *more* new business without
the usual added stenographic expense.
And speaking of new business,
those distinctive IBM letters are really
impressing prospects and boosting
our company prestige. Based on
performance, we're going 100% IBM!"

IBM ELECTRIC
TYPEWRITERS | . . . OUTSELL ALL OTHER ELECTRICS COMBINED!

©1955, International Business Machines Corp.

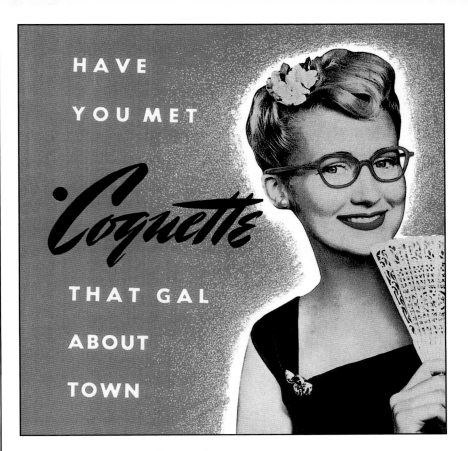

HAVE
YOU MET
Coquette
THAT GAL
ABOUT
TOWN

Left: The answer: one pair for the office...

Above: and another, for play. That's what
"specs appeal" is all about!

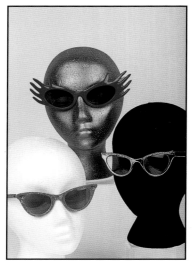

Chapter 3: "
MADE IN THE SHADE"

Sun Glasses Come Out Of The Shadows

Like millions of Americans, thousands of Brazilians wear and treasure Bausch & Lomb Ray-Ban sun glasses. Now, since the dedication this year of the ultra-modern U.S. Embassy building in Rio, the fame of the Ray-Ban name is evidenced still further. Among the architectural features of the lush 12-story structure are its massive green glare-proof first floor windows, which are of virtually the same hue as Ray-Ban lenses. Hence, and in true Brazilian humor, the natives have dubbed the Embassy building "Edifico Ray-Ban."
—*Balco News*
November-December, 1953

Even without "Edifico Ray-Ban," sun glasses in the 1950s and '60s would still have been huge. Although colored lenses first came into vogue in the 1700s, it wasn't until the mid-twentieth century that "shades" really emerged as fashion choices for the masses. Sun glasses had previously been promoted for their prescriptive value—to protect against what American Optical ominously called "the infra-red heat rays that create strain and burning sensation in your eyes." By the late 1930s, however, their streamlined stylings were attracting a wider audience. Ray-Ban "aviators," for instance, were originally designed to be worn by Air Force fighter pilots. Hollywood liked the look, and beginning in the 1940s, stars of every magnitude were sporting these, as well as countless other Ray-Ban styles. Big, dark sun glasses were supposed to supply stars with welcome anonymity, but the actual result was the opposite. Sun glasses *attracted* attention. They were mysterious. They were alluring. They invited second looks. And, as the rest of America quickly realized, if Hollywood stars looked that good in them, think what they could do for ordinary folks!

With regular glasses, there were design limits: too extreme and they just wouldn't work at the office. With sun glasses, worn primarily for fun or for fashion, those limits disappeared. Sun glasses still had to keep out the sun. But more importantly, according to the ads, they had to "bewitch," "flatter," and be "the chic-est thing in eye fashion." Sun glasses were no longer just for sunny days. As Foster Grant promos proudly pro-

claimed, "you'll see almost as many at midnight in January as you will at high noon in July. "

Soon, the very stars wearing sun glasses to avoid recognition were promoting them to the rest of us. A Grantly ad featuring actress Hedy Lamarr reassured buyers that "fair Hollywood says a sun glass wardrobe's the latest thing." Wear Grantlys, and you could be as captivating as Hedy. Or, some years later, you could "hide behind those Foster Grants," and be as cosmopolitan as Peter Sellers, shown "under the heady influence of six of the season's hottest styles." Of course sun glasses were still, as Bausch & Lomb noted, "scientifically designed to keep your eyes cool, calm, and protected." But as the same ad noted, every Ray-Ban wearer was a "beauty with brains," whose "enchanting air makes heads turn." Which claim do you think sold more sun glasses?

The vintage sun glasses shown here represent the diversity of styles available mid-century, from both domestic and foreign manufacturers. They range from the extreme and highly decorative shapes popular in the 1950s to the oversize "wide-screen" frames and wraparounds that won approval in the '60s. Because sun glasses were (and remain) so popular, many were produced, and many affordably-priced pairs can still be found at flea markets, and shops specializing in period fashion accessories. Designer frames or unusual shapes may prove more expensive, but as an ad for Polaroid "C'Bon's" put it, "you'll be glad to pay the difference when you see the difference."

The fun of owning vintage sun glasses is, of course, in the wearing. Before donning your latest treasure, here are a few things to keep in mind:

- Older sun glasses may not have UV-coated lenses. If ultraviolet rays are a concern, have the lenses replaced.
- If the original sun glass lenses are prescription, replace them, or prepare for blurry days ahead.
- Wear with care: older glass lenses may not be shatterproof.
- Scratch, scratch: vintage plastic lenses are susceptible to almost-impossible-to-remove scratches.
- Stumble on just the right frame, but the lenses are clear? That's easy: have the original lenses replaced with dark ones. The result? Instant sun glasses!
- Go for comfort: you're wearing them for pleasure, right? So they'd better be a pleasant fit.
- When it comes to sun glasses, cat-eyes *are* for everyone. You're not wearing them 'round the clock, and hidden behind those dark lenses, you'll see yourself in a new light!

Behind this international boom in sun glasses lies a phenomenon that fascinates psychologists and taxi drivers alike: the unmistakable personality change that begins to take place the moment anyone gets behind a pair of these tinted marvels. From Balboa Beach to Biarritz, everyone is wearing "shades."
—Foster Grant ad, 1964

Top left: Is it the sun glasses or is it the plunging neckline? Either way, this Bausch & Lomb executive looks pleased to crown Nancy Ann Miller as "Miss Specs Appeal of 1953!"

Center left: This 1956 flyer for American Optical Company's "Calobar" sun glasses stressed their therapeutic value. Calobars not only reduced glare but also "gave an actual cooling sensation to the eyes!"

Bottom left: Flyer reverse.

Right: Sun glasses provide an instant touch of mystery and glamour for this August, 1946 *McCall's* cover girl. Her photographer seems to agree!

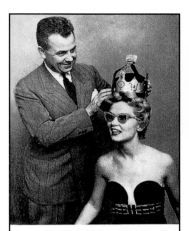

FRAME SALES chief Dick Eisenhart crowns contest winner Nancy Ann Miller as "Miss Specs Appeal of 1953."

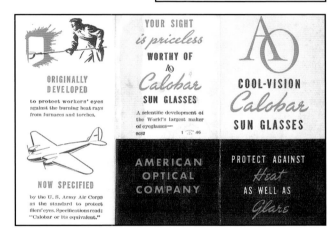

ORIGINALLY DEVELOPED
to protect workers' eyes against the burning heat rays from furnaces and torches.

NOW SPECIFIED
by the U. S. Army Air Corps as the standard to protect fliers' eyes. Specifications read: "Calobar or its equivalent."

YOUR SIGHT *is priceless* WORTHY OF

AO *Calobar* SUN GLASSES

A scientific development of the World's largest maker of eyeglasses.

AO COOL-VISION *Calobar* SUN GLASSES

AMERICAN OPTICAL COMPANY

PROTECT AGAINST *Heat* AS WELL AS *Glare*

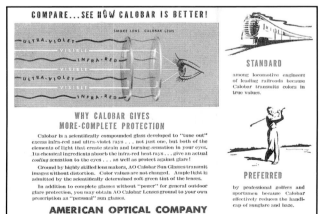

COMPARE...SEE HOW CALOBAR IS BETTER!

WHY CALOBAR GIVES MORE-COMPLETE PROTECTION

Calobar is a scientifically compounded glass developed to "tune out" excess infra-red and ultra-violet rays . . . not just one, but both of the elements of light that create strain and burning sensation in your eyes. Its chemical ingredients absorb the infra-red heat rays . . . give an actual *cooling sensation to the eyes* . . . as well as protect against glare!

Ground by highly skilled lens makers, AO Calobar Sun Glasses transmit images without distortion. Color values are not changed. Ample light is admitted by the scientifically determined soft green tint of the lenses.

In addition to complete glasses without "power" for general outdoor glare protection, you may obtain AO Calobar Lenses ground to your own prescription as "personal" sun glasses.

AMERICAN OPTICAL COMPANY

STANDARD
among locomotive engineers of leading railroads because Calobar transmits colors in true values.

PREFERRED
by professional golfers and sportsmen because Calobar effectively reduces the handicap of sunglare and haze.

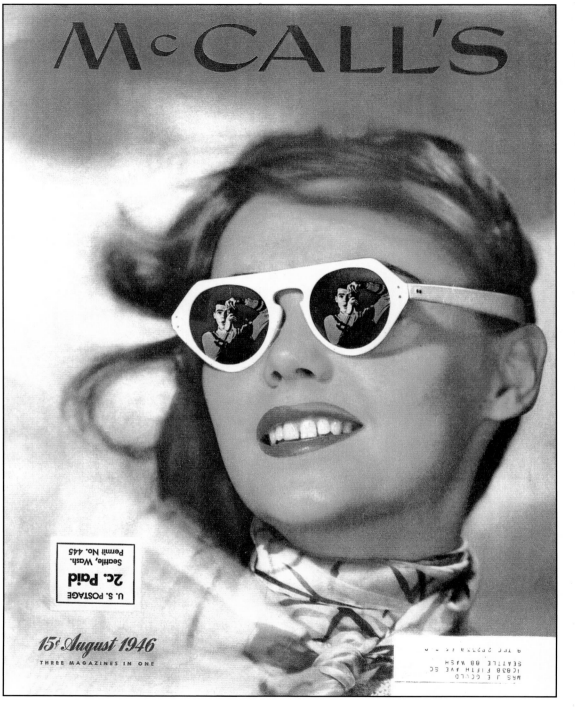

McCALL'S

15¢ August 1946
THREE MAGAZINES IN ONE

U. S. POSTAGE
2c. Paid
Seattle, Wash.
Permit No. 445

MRS J E GOULD
1083B FIFTH AVE SC
SEATTLE 88 WASH

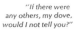
"If there were any others, my dove, would I not tell you?"

Isn't that Peter Sellers behind those Foster Grants?

(The very same, currently starring in the United Artists film "A Shot in the Dark")

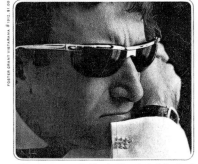
FOSTER GRANT VISTARAMA #1912, $1.00

"Come now, croupier! Surely this pathetic little pile of chips can't be the entire bank at Monte Carlo..."

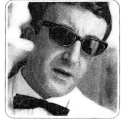
FOSTER GRANT DEMI AMBER #3603, $2.98

"My good Fritz, you can hardly hang a key around a busboy's neck and expect to come up with a wine steward."

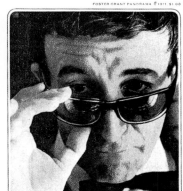
FOSTER GRANT PANORAMA #1911, $1.00

"Ravishing, my dear, but aren't you likely to catch cold or something?"

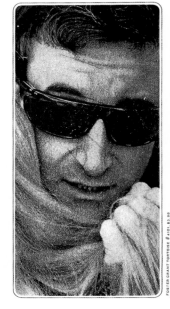
FOSTER GRANT TORTOISE #4101, $3.98

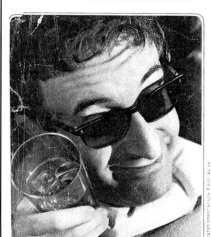
FOSTER GRANT NYLON #2001, $2.98

...et me put it this way—if it were not for her money, I should probably have made something quite splendid of myself."

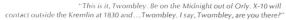
"This is it, Twombley. Be on the Midnight out of Orly. X-10 will contact outside the Kremlin at 1830 and...Twombley, I say, Twombley, are you there?"

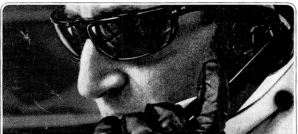

IT'S getting harder and harder to tell an old friend from a mysterious stranger. From Balboa Beach to Biarritz, everyone is wearing "shades". What's more, you'll see almost as many at midnight in January as you will at high noon in July.

Behind this international boom in sunglasses lies a phenomenon that fascinates psychologists and taxi drivers alike: the unmistakable personality change that begins to take place the moment anyone gets behind a pair of these tinted marvels.

Peter Sellers demonstrates. Normally quiet and unassuming, here you see him under the heady influence of six of the season's hottest styles from Foster Grant, world's largest maker of sunglasses.

Popularly-priced Foster Grants combine the best of both worlds—European fashion and American technology. And their ff77 lenses meet rigid U. S. standards for eye protection that many of even the most expensive imports don't.

If Sellers' reactions are any clue, millions of men and women who slip behind a pair of Foster Grants for the first time this summer will be seeing themselves in a new light.

© FOSTER GRANT, LEOMINSTER, MASS.

No celebrities here, just an appeal to the teen market. "Goin' Steady" sun glasses by Foster Grant.

"Who's that hiding behind those Foster Grants?" The sun glass manufacturer's popular ad campaign featured various celebrities wearing the company's product. Here, Peter Sellers gets the Foster Grant treatment, circa 1964.

66

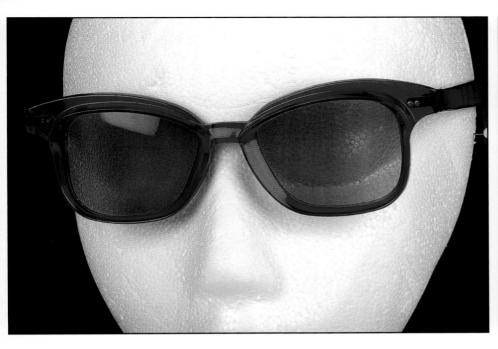

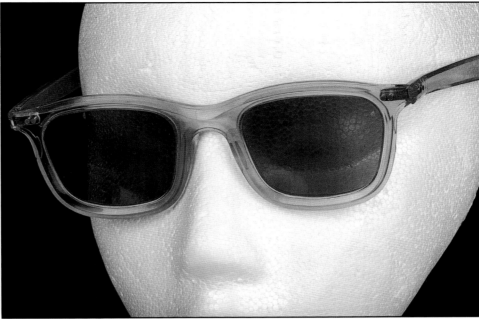

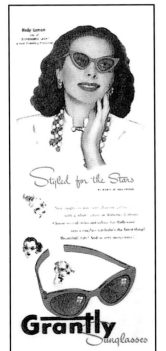

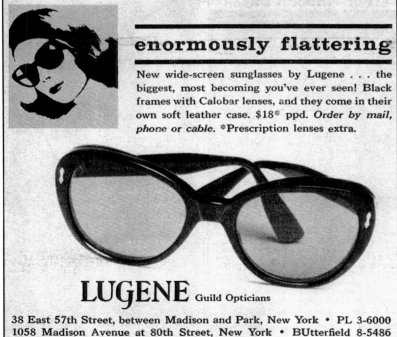

Top left: These clear red shades are by Grantly. $45-55.

Top right: Also by Grantly, squarish sun glasses in clear pink. $45-55.

Bottom left: Another celebrity heard from. Grantly's "Styled for the Stars" ad features screen queen Hedy Lamarr.

Bottom right: "The biggest, most becoming sun glasses you've ever seen." A 1962 ad for the "wide-screen" model by Lugene.

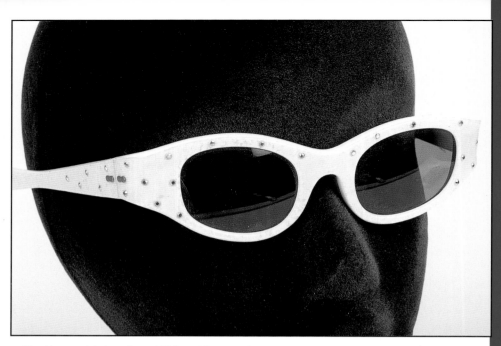

This May model dates from 1958, and features rhinestone studs on pearlized plastic. $110-125.

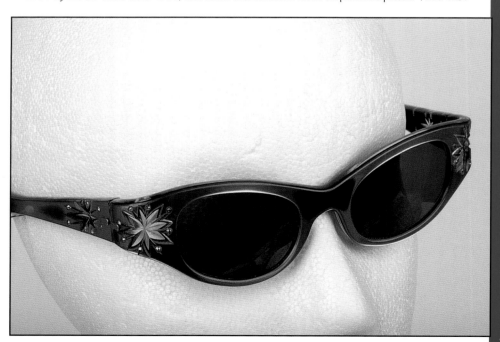

May-time once more: silver and smoke with star cutaways, rhinestone accents. $110-125.

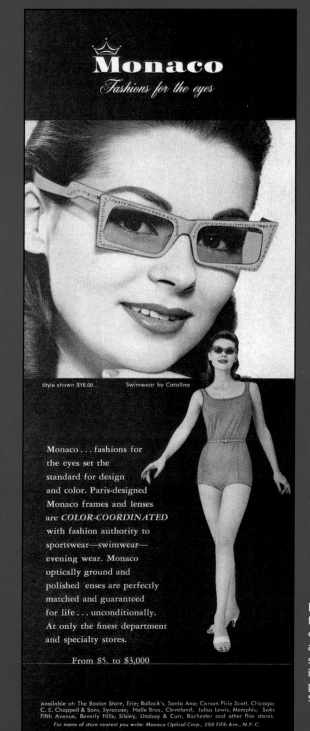
Here's an idea: sun glass frames and lenses "color-coordinated with fashion authority to sportswear—swimwear—evening wear." An innovation from Monaco, with prices ranging from $5—to $3,000! *Vogue*, May, 1962.

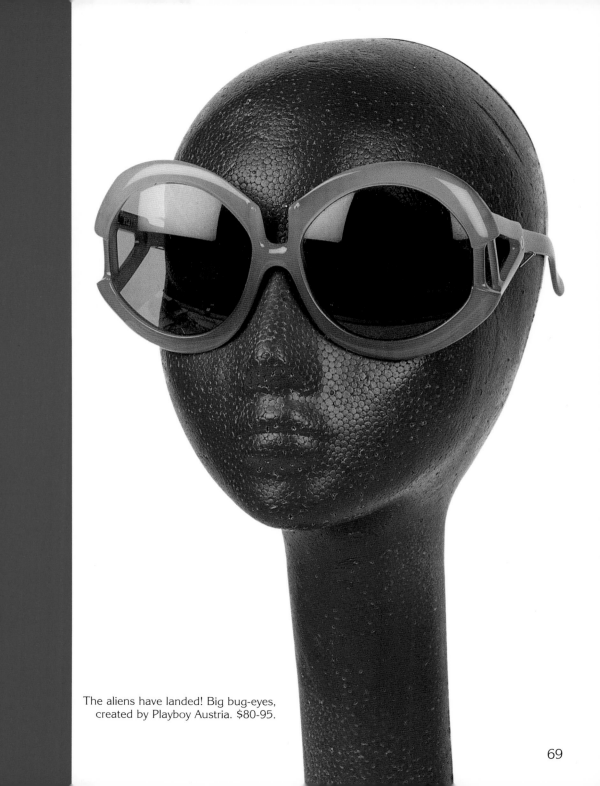

The aliens have landed! Big bug-eyes, created by Playboy Austria. $80-95.

69

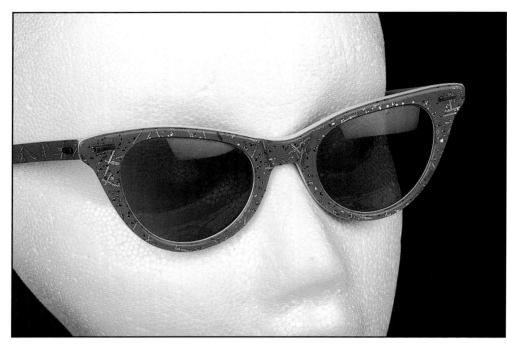

Sun glass sparkle: "Cool Ray Polaroids" in turquoise with glitter. $60-70.

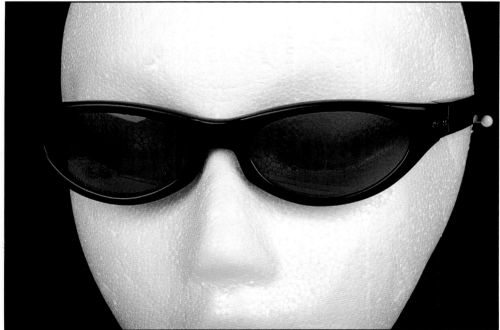

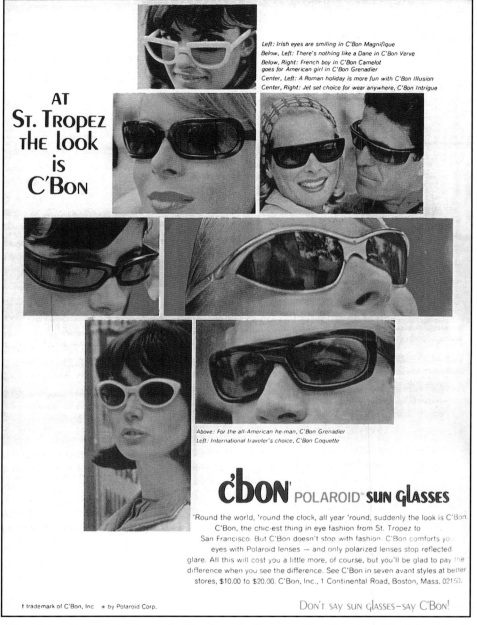

C'Bon, "the chic-est thing in eye fashion from St. Tropez to San Francisco." By Polaroid, of course, as advertised in *Vogue*, July, 1965.

Wraparound from Polaroid, in black. $60-70.

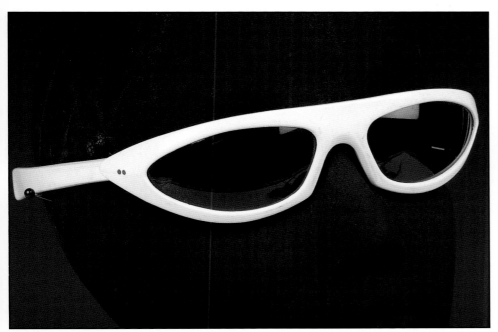

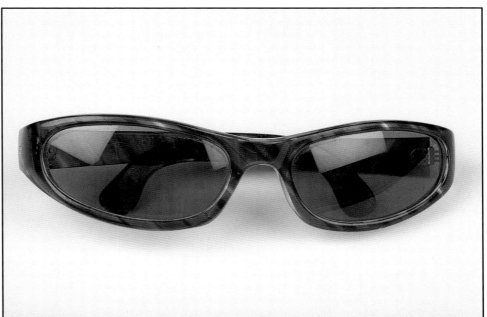

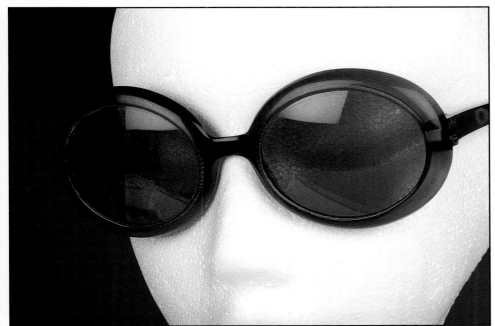

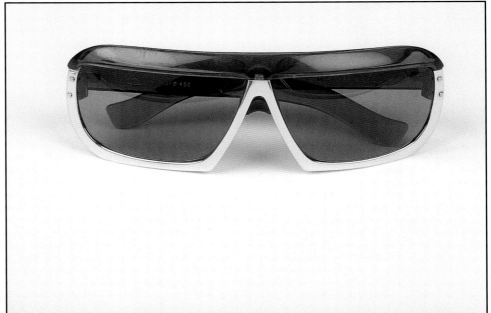

Top left: More wraps, these in white, and designed for Polaroid by "Cari Michelle." $60-70.

Top right: Also by "Cari Michelle" for Polaroid, brown wraps, $60-70.

Bottom left: The bugs are back: amber bug-eyes by Polaroid, $40-45.

Bottom right: Let's boogie! Amber and gold large disco shades by Polaroid. $50-60.

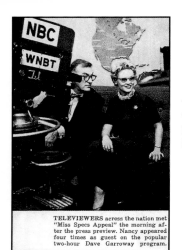

Those television lights must be bright. "Miss Specs Appeal 1953" dons her Bausch & Lomb Ray-Bans, for a TV interview with Dave Garroway.

TELEVIEWERS across the nation met "Miss Specs Appeal" the morning after the press preview. Nancy appeared four times as guest on the popular two-hour Dave Garroway program.

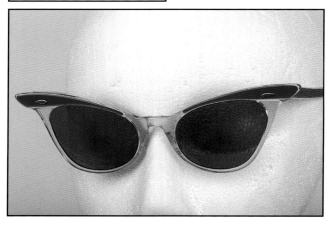

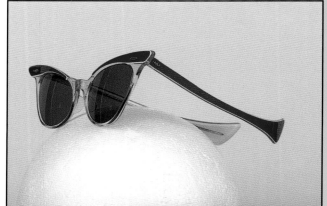

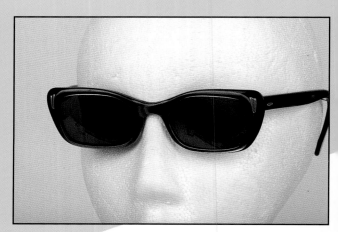

Left: Ready for flight: Ray-Ban "Red Wings." $60-70.

Center: "Red Wing" temple detail.

Right: The no-nonsense look. Ray-Ban "Pewter Squares." $70-85.

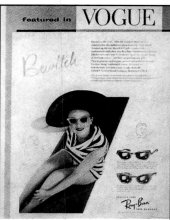

Want to "Bewitch?" It's a cinch with Ray-Bans, according to this B & L ad from 1955.

DISPLAY CARDS of the full-page color ads of Ray-Ban styles which will appear in the April 15 *Vogue* and May 28 *Saturday Evening Post*, will be a point-of-purchase aid.

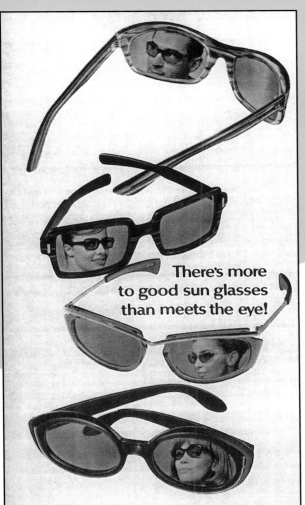

There's more
to good sun glasses
than meets the eye!

How smart you *look* in Ray-Ban Sun Glasses! There's an enchanting air about you that makes heads turn, gives you a very special place in the sun. Choose from dozens of frame styles so flattering they're almost wicked!

How smart you *are* in Ray-Bans. Lenses of optical glass are *scientifically* designed to keep your eyes cool, calm, and protected. Be a beauty with brains in Ray-Ban Sun Glasses. At optical offices and better stores. Wear glasses? You can have Ray-Bans in your prescription. For free style catalog, write Bausch & Lomb, Rochester, New York 14602.

BAUSCH & LOMB ⑲ *Ray-Ban* SUN GLASSES

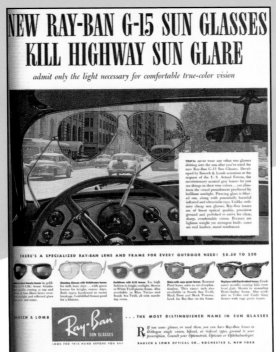

NEW RAY-BAN G-15 SUN GLASSES
KILL HIGHWAY SUN GLARE

admit only the light necessary for comfortable true-color vision

THERE'S A SPECIALIZED RAY-BAN LENS AND FRAME FOR EVERY OUTDOOR NEED! $8.50 TO $20

Ray-Ban
SUN GLASSES

... THE MOST DISTINGUISHED NAME IN SUN GLASSES

BAUSCH & LOMB OPTICAL CO., ROCHESTER 2, NEW YORK

Left: Still bewitchin': a Ray-Ban ad from *Vogue*, June, 1965. "How smart you look in Ray-Ban Sun Glasses. There's an enchanting air about you that makes heads turn, gives you a very special place in the sun." Mmm-hmmm.

Top right: Of course, there were practical considerations, too. This *Saturday Evening Post* ad from May 28, 1955 reminded buyers that Ray-Bans "eliminate the visual punishment produced by brilliant sunlight." Ouch!

Bottom: Bugs again, in blue. Bug-eyes by Renould. $80-95.

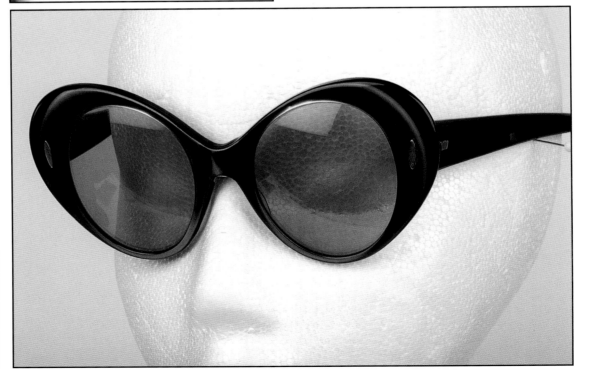

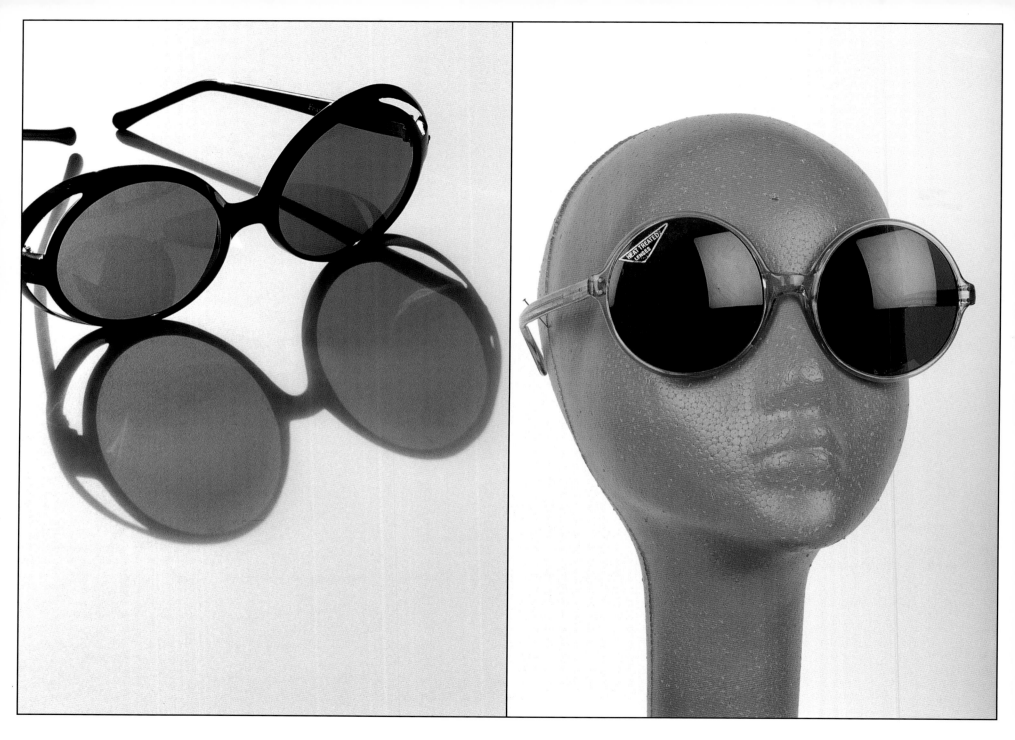

Opposite page:
Left: From Selecta, "#5560" in black. $55-65.

Right: The "Rondo" by Selecta. $55-65.

Also by Selecta, irregular egg-shape frames with temple cutouts. $55-65.

Selecta's "4000" in black. $55-65.

The "4000" again in White Pearl. $55-65.

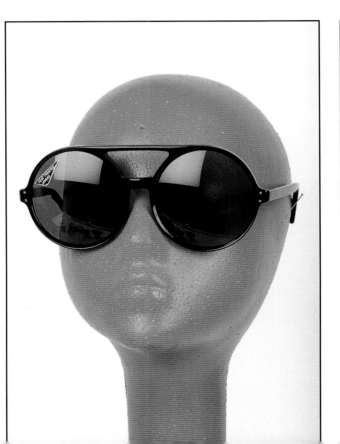

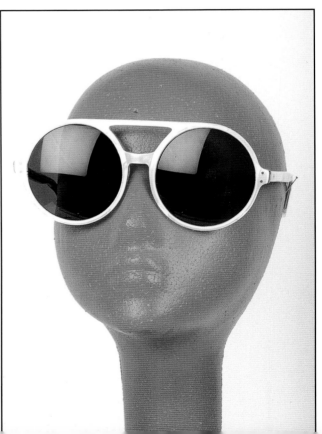

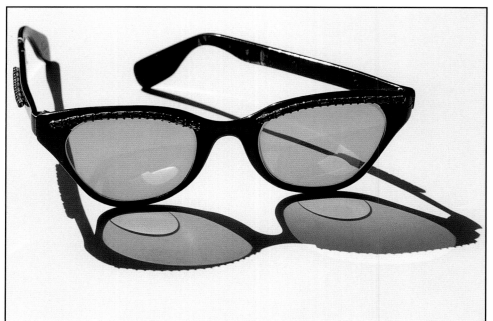

By Tura, dark blue with rectangular rhinestone trim and pale blue lenses. $130-140.

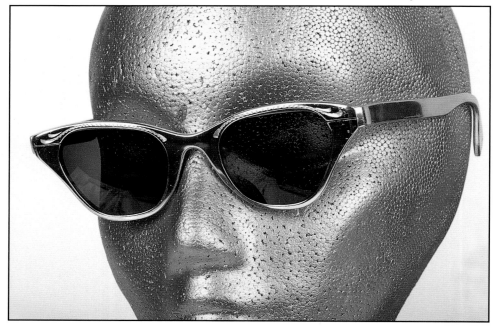

Another Tura, silvery with engraved brow design. $60-70.

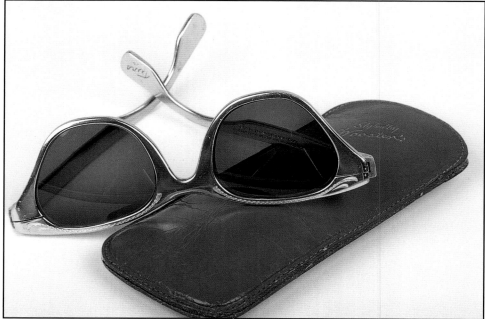

The same, with case.

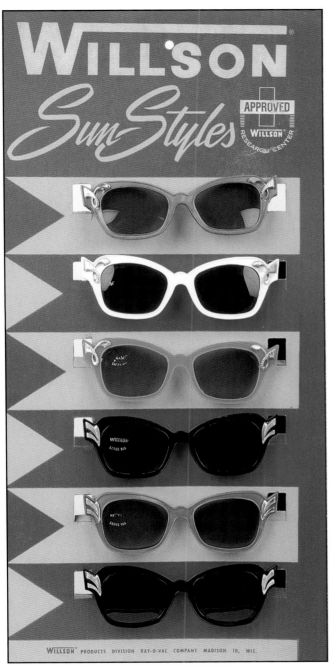

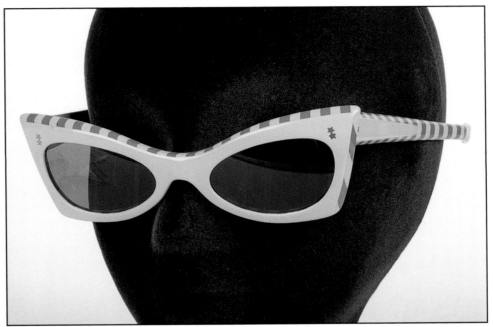

Display card for Willson Sun Styles by Ray-O-Vac (and you thought they only made batteries!)

From the early '50s, enticing "Suntimers" by Victory, in lime-green laminated plastic. $110-125.

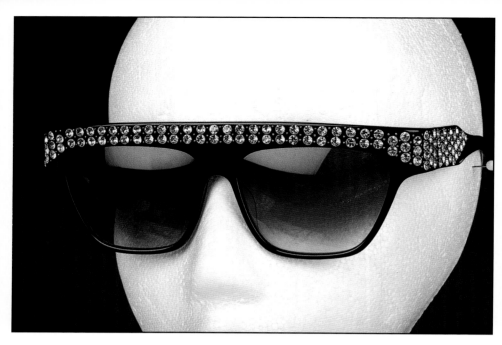

Think sunshine—think French Riviera. These French imports by "Anne Marie" feature a rhinestone 'unibrow'. $110-120.

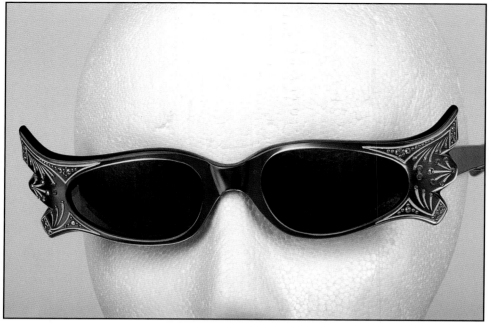

So exotic! So French! Triple-flare cat-eyes with rhinestones. $140-160.

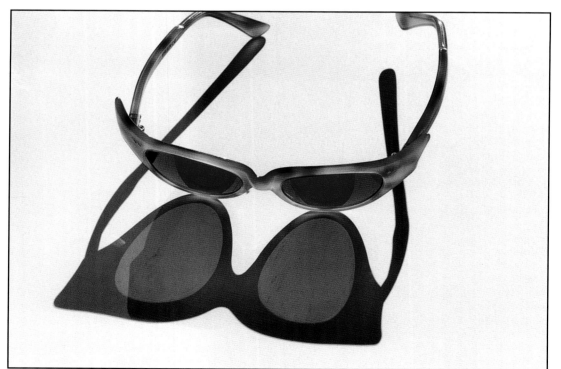

More cat-eyes, dating from Paris in the 1950s. $150-175.

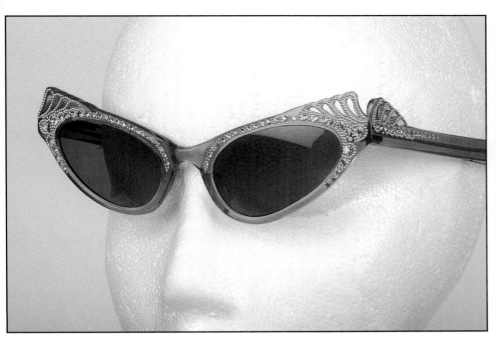

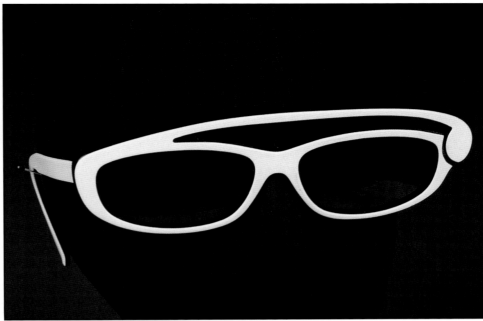

Also French, cutaways in clear pink, with applied granular silver ball decor. $140-160.

Fore! From Paris by Chantel Thomas, this sporty pair features a golf club cutout above the brow. $100-110.

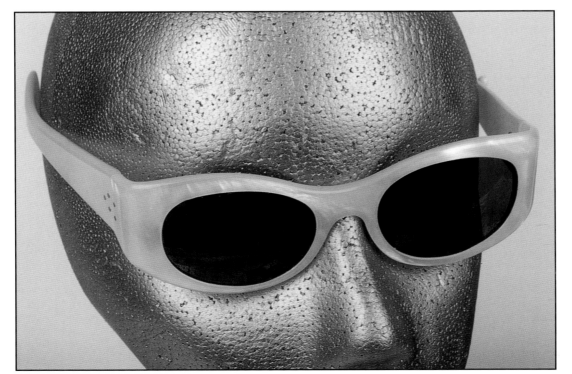

French, by ER: white pearlized frames with extra-width temples. $80-95.

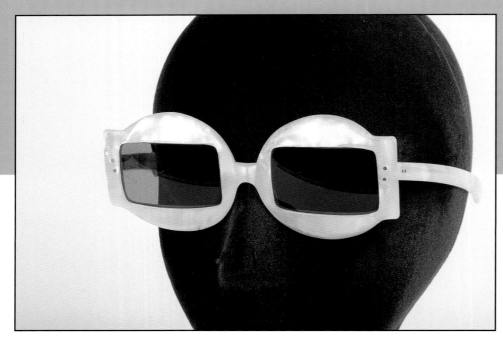

Squaring the circles: geometric white pearlized design by Frame France, $120-130.

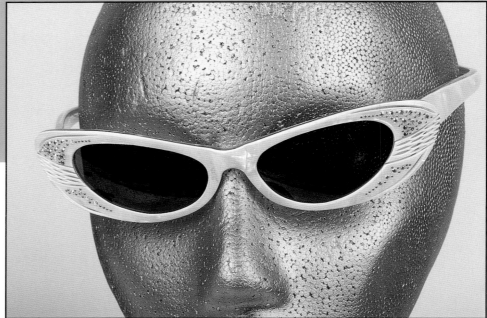

Meow! White cat-eye sun glasses from France. The frames feature a white mesh cutaway pattern, highlighted with rhinestones. $120-135.

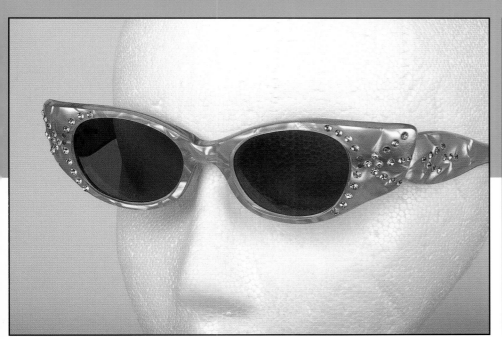

Mamma mia! A spicy pink marbleized pair from sunny Italy. $90-110.

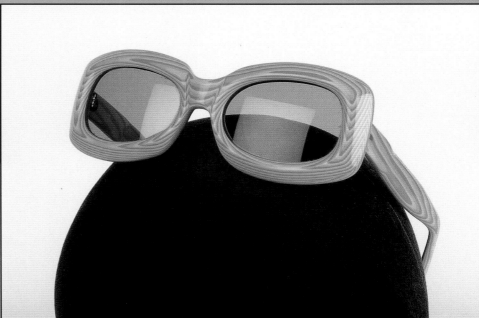

Italian wood-grain "picture frames," by Ritmo. $75-125.

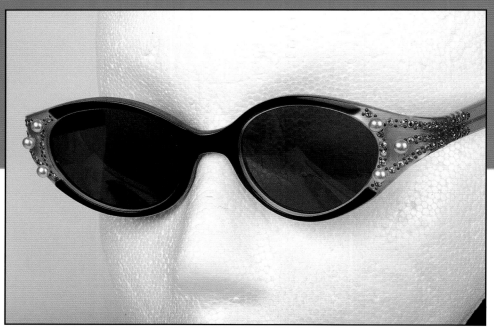

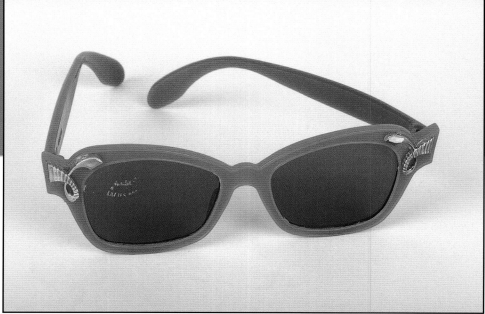

Let's face it, some sun glasses simply radiate "specs appeal." Our sampler of '50s and '60s look-at-me favorites begins with a midnight blue overlay on pearl, with pearl and rhinestone trim. $100-115.

Hot fun in the summertime! An orangey-red attention-getter, with silver brow accents. $45-55.

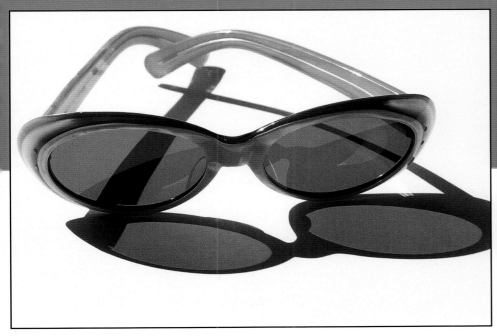

Cool pink laminates. $60-70.

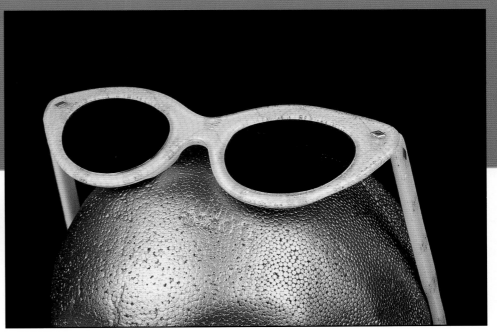

Sleek white, with silver-gold netting. $95-110.

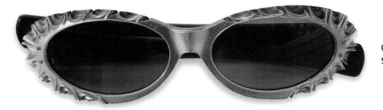

Gold, with multicolored carved rims.
$90-100.

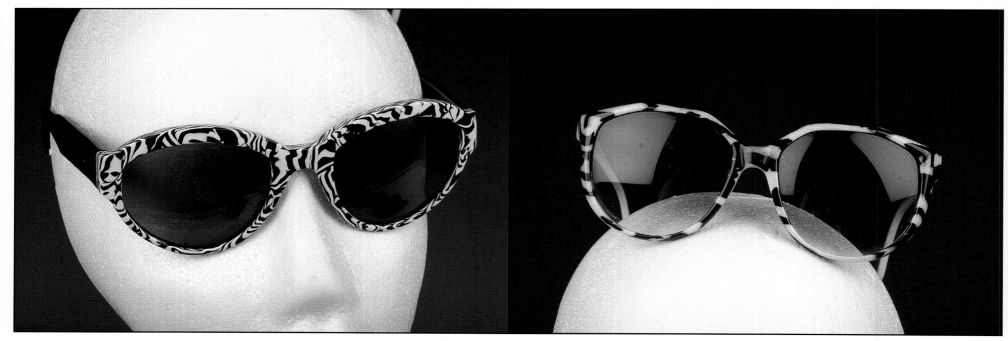

Jungle fever: zebra-pattern frames, black temples. $60-70.

Continuing the zebra stampede: oversize squarish frames, white temples. $60-70.

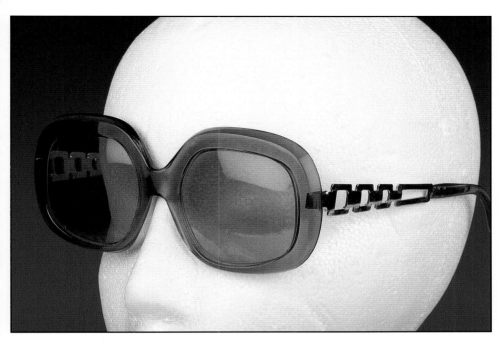

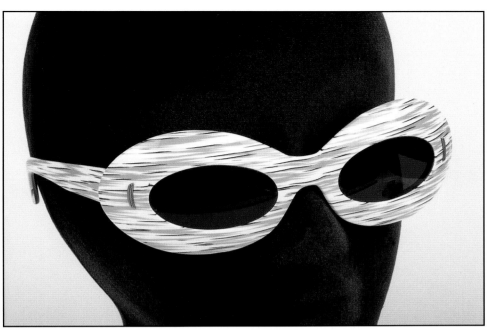

To the 21st century and beyond! Futuristic amber frames, with a squarish form echoed in the temple design. $90-110.

"Suntimer" in pink, black, and white laminated plastic. Early 1960s. $110-125.

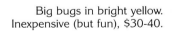

Big bugs in bright yellow. Inexpensive (but fun), $30-40.

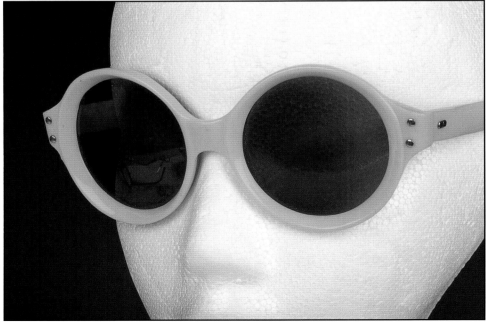

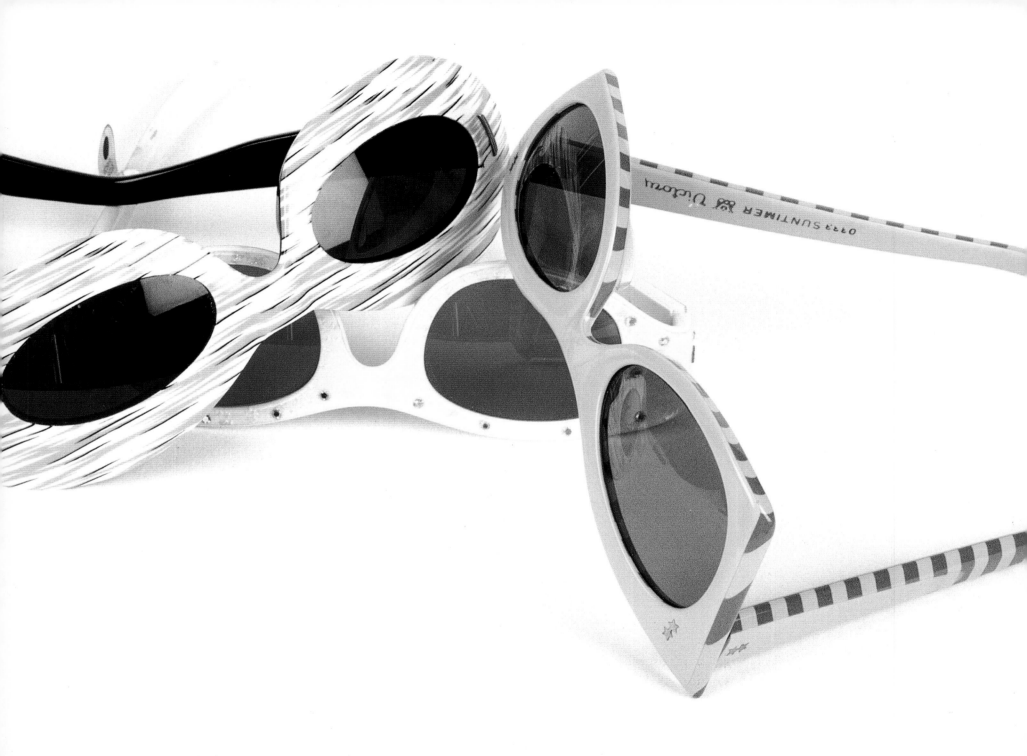

THE *Stoco* ASTIG GOGGLE

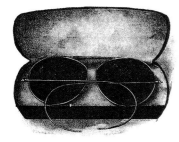

The *Stoco* Astig Goggle will fit any face perfectly and comfortably without any adjustment whatever. This is accomplished by the bar spring design and the form of the lenses which are so shaped as to follow closely the contour of the face. Your customers will appreciate the comfort and protection features of the *Stoco* Astig Goggle.

The frame including the Velvet Tip temples is 1-10 12 K gold filled throughout. The deeply curved 52 x 43 mm. coquille lenses are furnished in assorted shades of amber and fieuzal. Each Astig Goggle is packed in a good quality self-closing case.

Price........$24.00 per dozen

STANDARD OPTICAL CO.

Geneva, N. Y.

Just right for a spin in the Model T! The Stoco "Astig Goggle," "furnished in assorted shades of amber and fieuzal," as advertised in *The Western Optical World*, April, 1918.

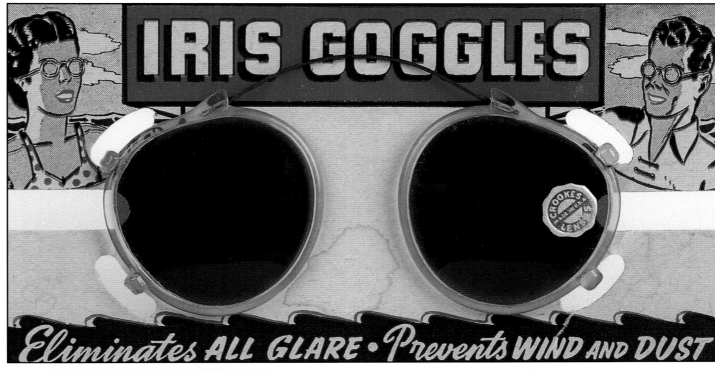

Something else to goggle at: the "Iris Goggles," guaranteed to "eliminate all glare—prevent wind and dust."

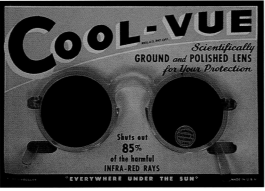

"Cool-Vue," available "everywhere under the sun."

Opposite page:
Good day, sunshine! An eye-catching sun glass selection guaranteed to chase the clouds away.

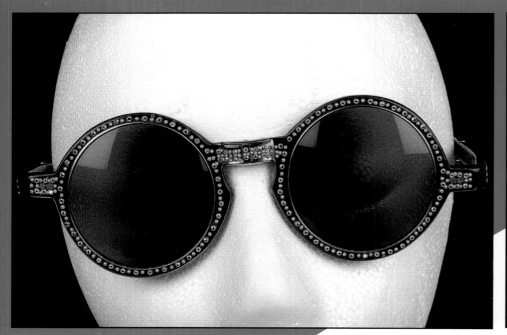

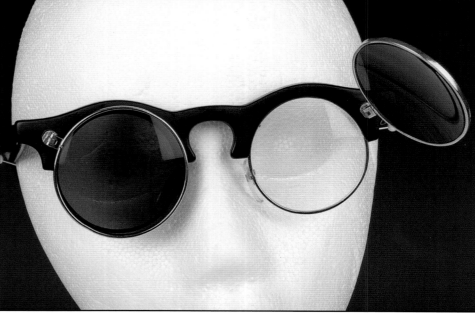

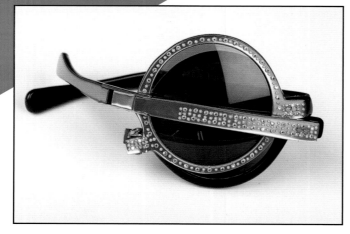

Top left: Elegant, and compact too! Rhinestone-covered folding sun glasses from Japan. $130-150.

Bottom left: The same, all folded up and ready to go.

Right: Use them when you need them: safety glasses with flip-down shades. $45-50.

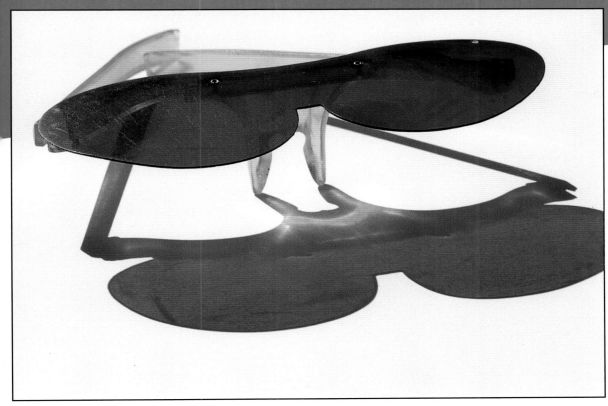

It only looks like a grasshopper: flip-up visor sun glasses, with green lenses on amber frames. $40-50.

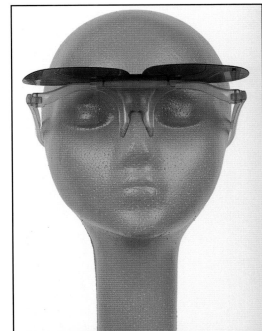

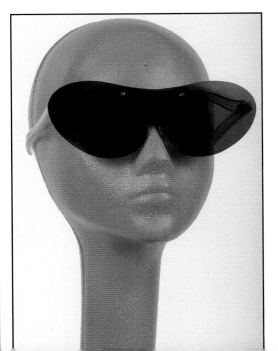

Left: Up, they're a visor...

Right: ...and down, they're shades!

89

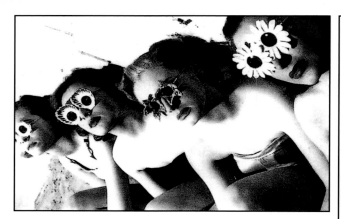

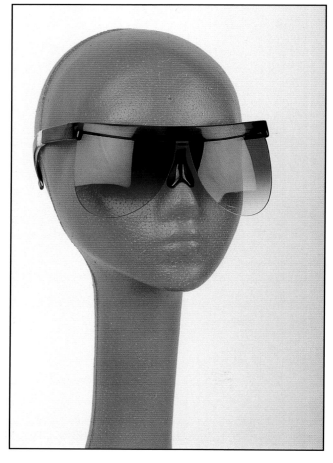

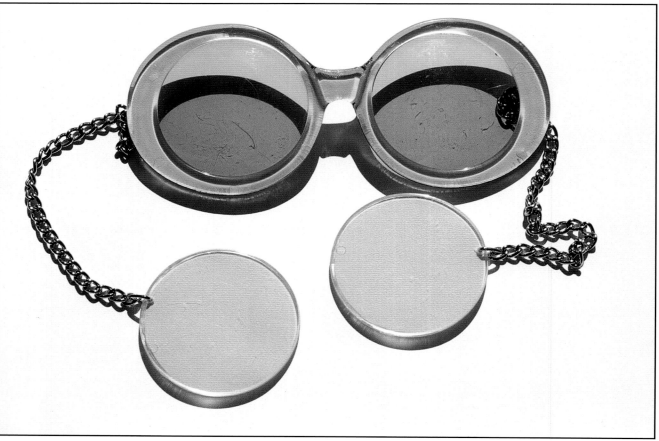

From the sensational '60s: who needs temples? Earring chains are so much more "with it!" $120-160.

Top left: From the 1950s: sun glass styles that defy description, not for the faint-of-heart!

Bottom left: Every man wants a pair: Italian oversize men's futuristic sun glasses, with lenses hanging from brow. $80-90.

From the 1990s: retro reigns! $20-30 each.

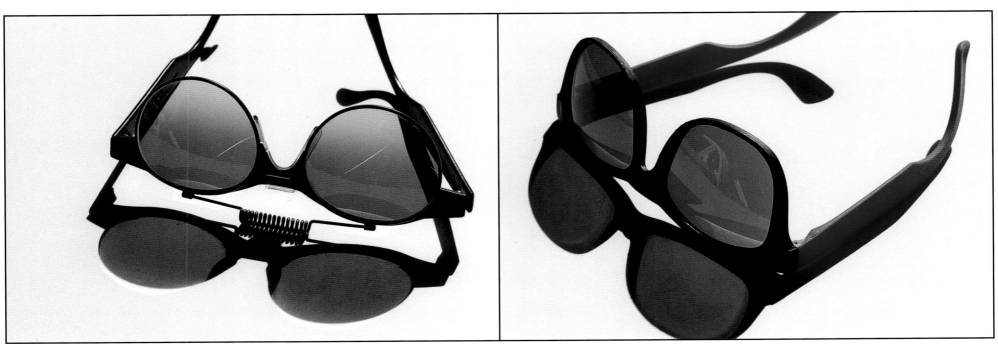

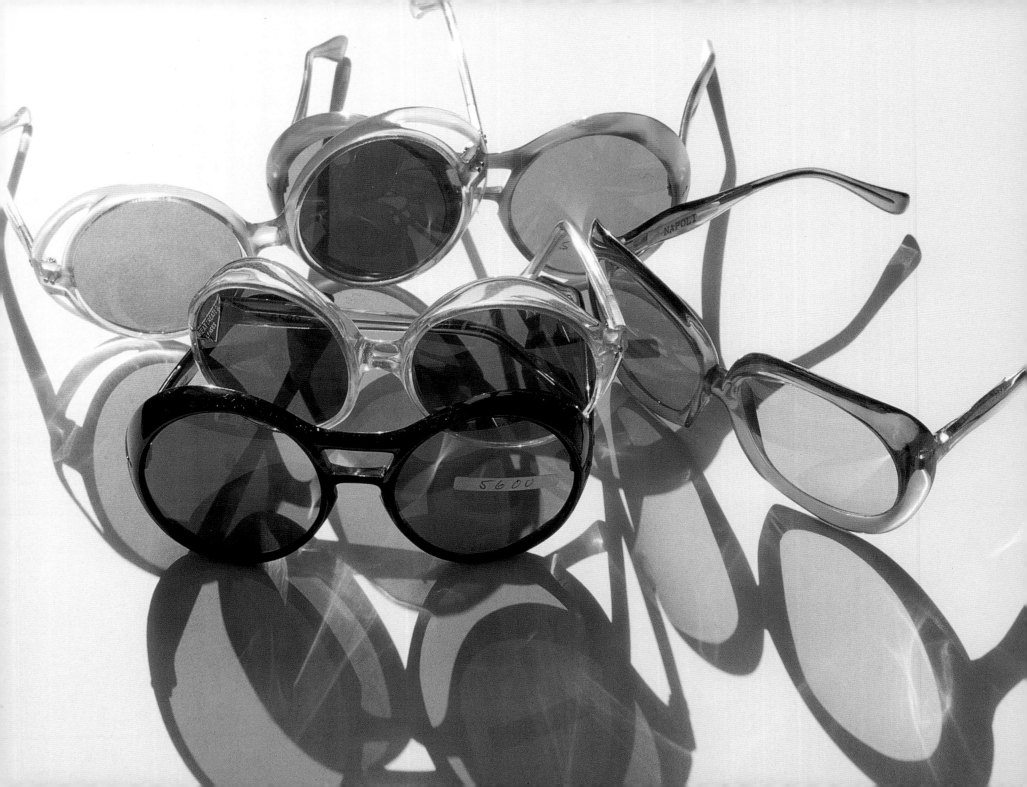

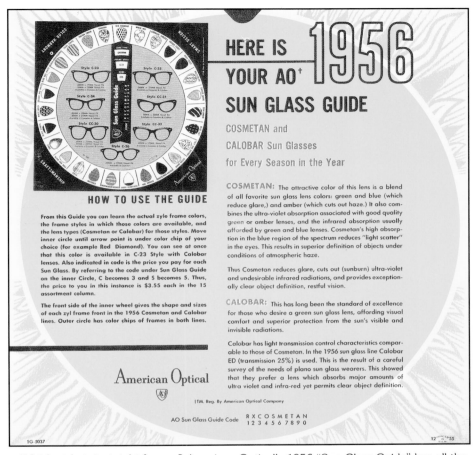

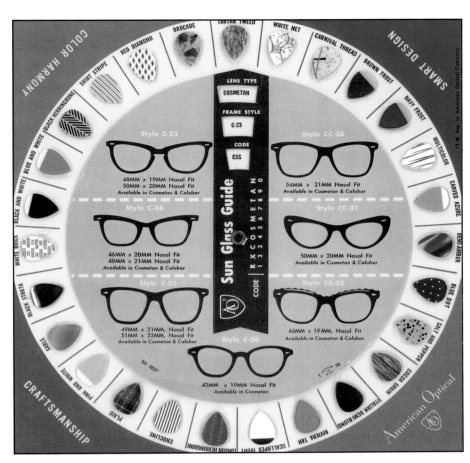

Which style is just right for you? American Optical's 1956 "Sun Glass Guide" has all the answers!

The "Guide" in all its glory. Break out the Coppertone and celebrate!

Opposite page:
"I only count the sunny hours." Sun glass display by Selecta.

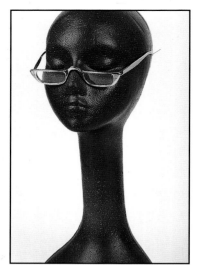

Chapter 4:

"SIGHT FOR SORE EYES"

A Variety Of Vision Helpers

The same convexity of glass through which a man sees clearest and best at the distance properly for reading is not the best for greater distances. I therefore had formerly two pair of glasses which I shifted occasionally. I had the glasses cut, and half of each associated in the same circle. By this means I have only to move my eyes up or down, the proper glasses always being ready.
—Benjamin Franklin, 1784

All right, admit it: you wear them "just for reading." Or "just to see the prices on menus." Or "just for close work." Or " just for..." (fill in the blank).

Vanity is always with us, and mid-twentieth century manufacturers provided plenty of eyewear options for "part-timers," those who didn't yet need (or hadn't yet admitted needing) glasses on a full-time basis. Included in this chapter are various vision aids, from hand-held magnifiers and lorgnettes to half-glasses, makeup glasses, and (for the really vain, but desperate) fold-away models. When it came to discreetly assisting the semi-visually impaired, '50s and '60s manufacturers had an inventive eye. Mr. Franklin would be proud.

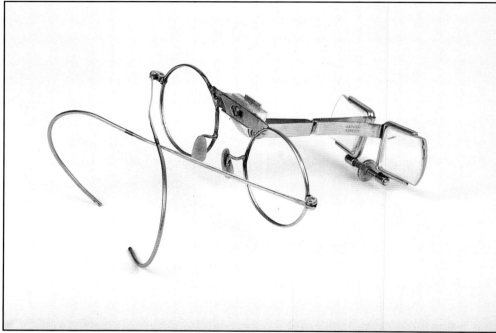

The next step: magnifiers, when the reading glass just won't work the way it used to. This pair has adjustable front magnifying lenses. $60-70.

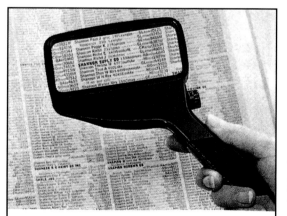

ILLUMINATED reading glass is the first to go on sale in the United States.

The first sign: the "illuminated reading glass," handy for those days when they seem to be making the type smaller. A 1954 vision helper from Bausch & Lomb.

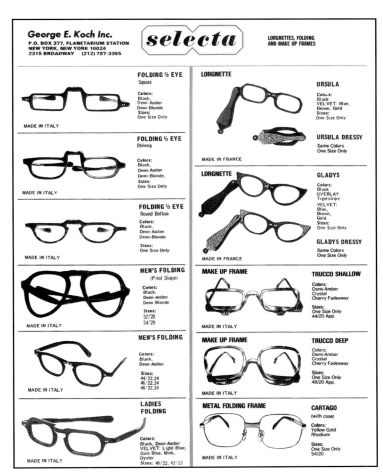

Top left: Once you've accepted the inevitable, a whole host of options await. Here are some from Selecta.

Bottom left: Giving in at last: bifocals, for those days when the horizon gets awfully hazy. 1920s bifocal advertisement for H.J. Stead Optical Co.

Top right: The fashionable alternative to reading glasses: the lorgnette. In black with rhinestones, $70-80.

Bottom right: A London lorgnette from the 1920s. $200-225.

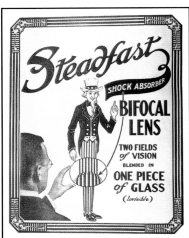

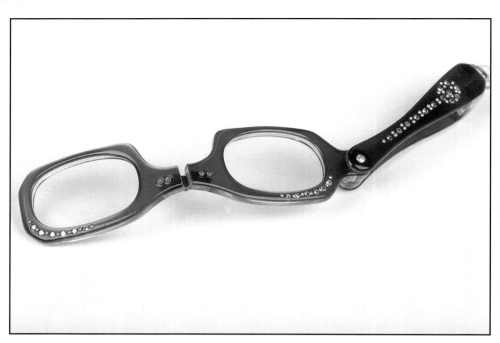

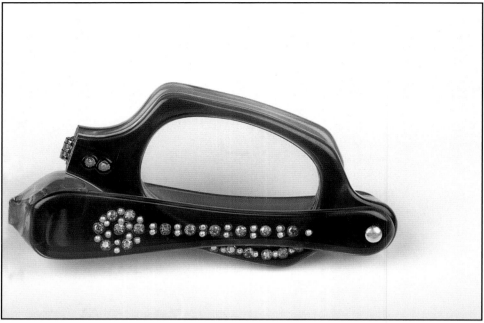

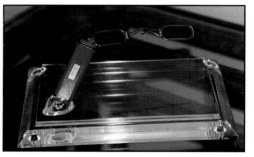

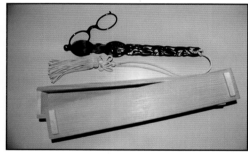

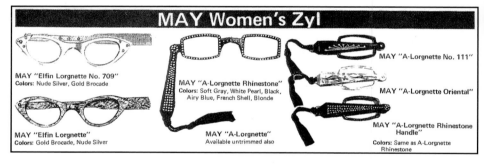

Top left: A lorgnette in light blue with rhinestones. $70-80.

Top right: The same, folded carefully away.

Bottom left: Lorgnette with red handle, from the estate of the Duchess of Windsor. The plaque monogram is "W.W." (Wallis Windsor)

Bottom center: Another historic lorgnette, this with carved tortoiseshell handle and white tassel, complete with carry box.

Bottom right: More modern lorgnettes: a selection from May, circa 1972.

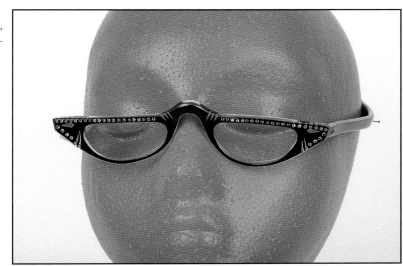

The "Cary Simili" by Selecta, in black. $65-75.

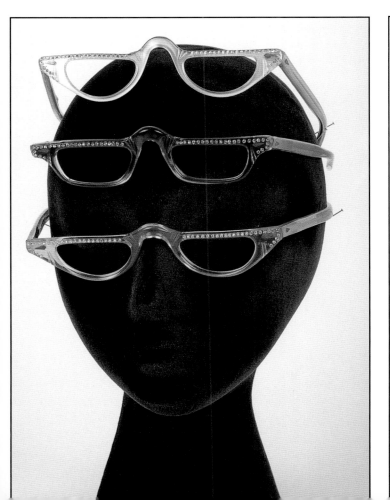

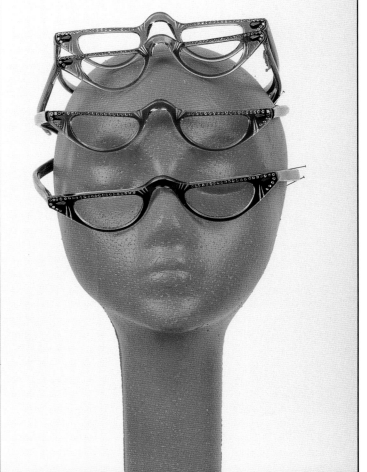

Left: Ready for the readers? This Selecta assortment of half-glasses includes the "Cary Simili" at top and bottom, the "Fairview Simili" at center. $65-75 each.

Right: A "Cary Simili" color assortment. $65-75 each.

97

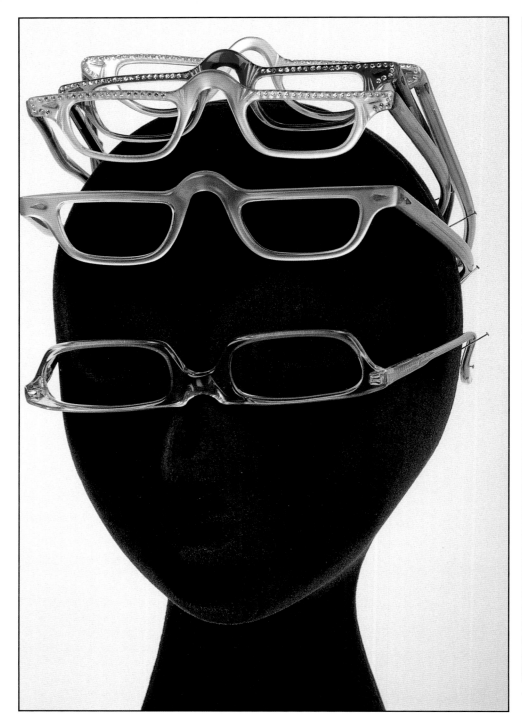

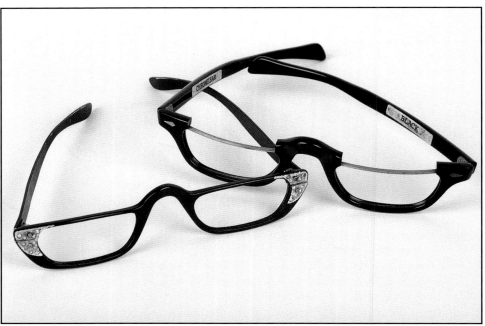

Rhinestoned readers at left, joined by the less showy "Fairview Crystal Bar" at right. $55-65 each.

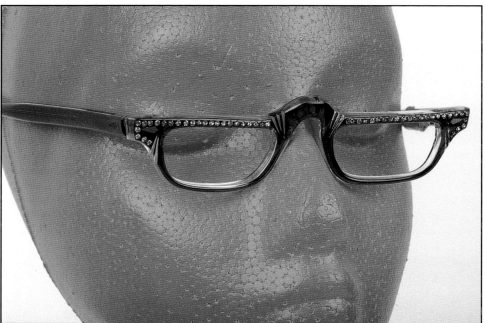

The "Fairview Simili" in Kelly Green Overlay. $65-75.

With rhinestones or without? The top three pairs are "Fairview Simili," with an unadorned "Fairview" below, and more traditional readers at bottom. "Simili," $65-75; plain, $55-65.

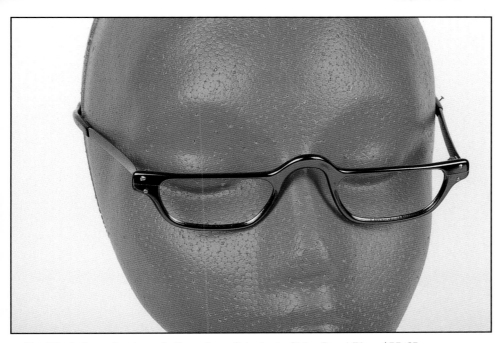

The "Scala," an aluminum half-eye from Selecta, in Shiny Royal Blue. $55-65.

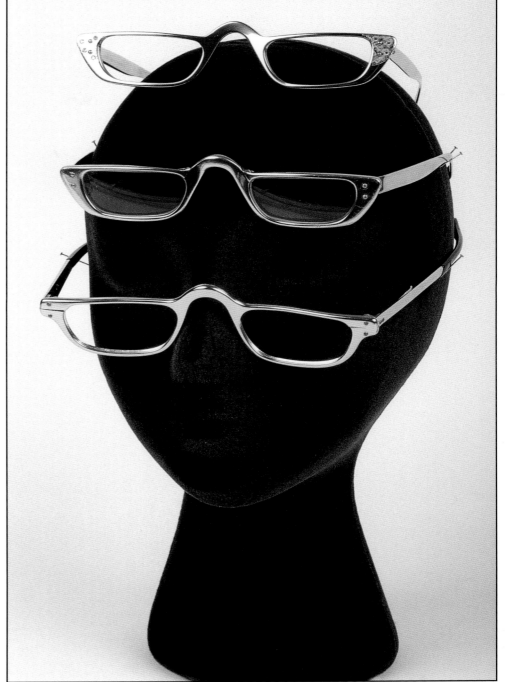

Three metallic readers. The bottom pair is Selecta "Scala" in Shiny Gold. $55-65 each.

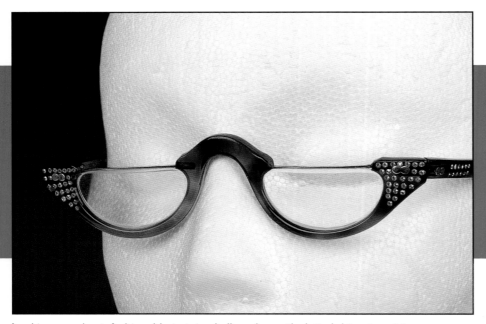

Looking your best: fashionable tortoiseshell readers with dotted rhinestone trim.

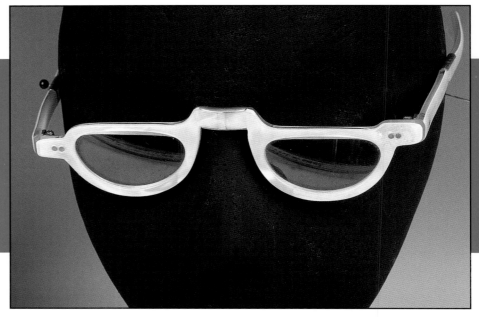

Pearl readers, $50-60.

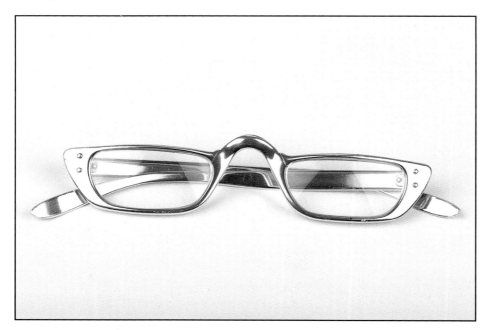

Aluminum readers, $30-40.

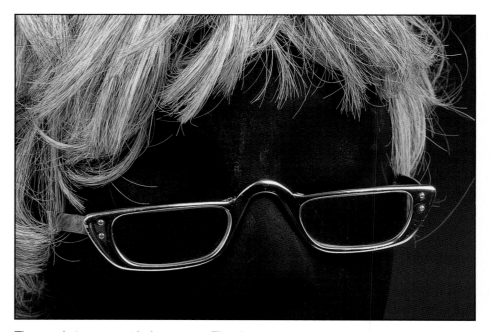

The gray hair comes with the territory. The aluminum readers again, doing their duty.

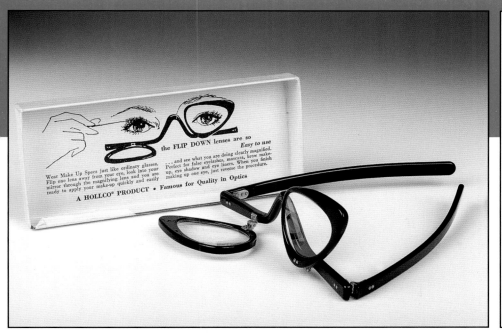

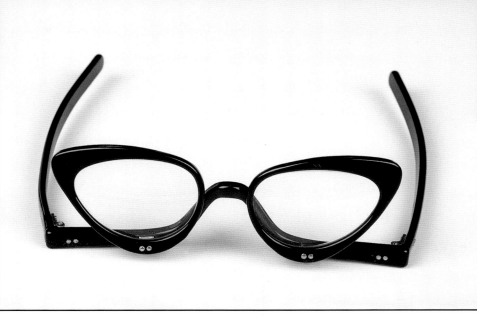

The "Flip Down Lenses" by Hollco. $65-75.

Hollco called these the "Flip Down Lenses." Included was the perhaps unnecessary instruction, "when you finish making up one eye, just reverse the procedure."

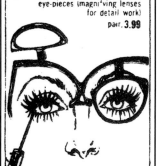

Another mascara brush in the eye? Reach for your "Flip-Up Make-Up Glasses," and put those eyelashes back where they belong!

101

Selecta's version, the "Trucco Shallow Make Up Frame" in Demi-Amber. $50-60.

The "Trucco Shallow" in Crystal. $50-60.

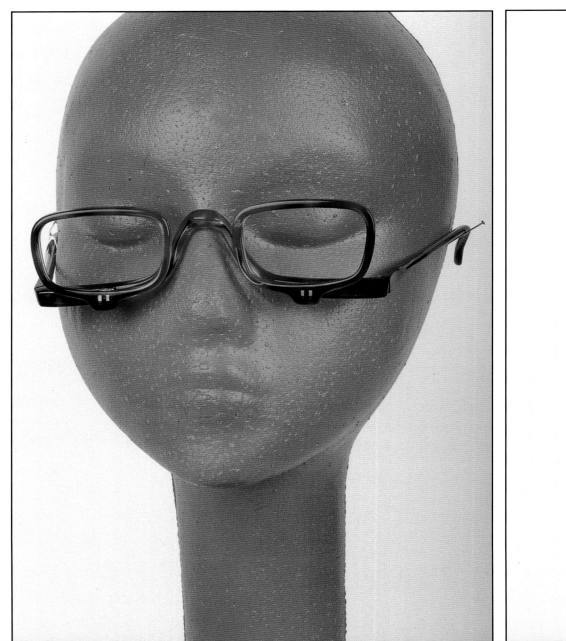

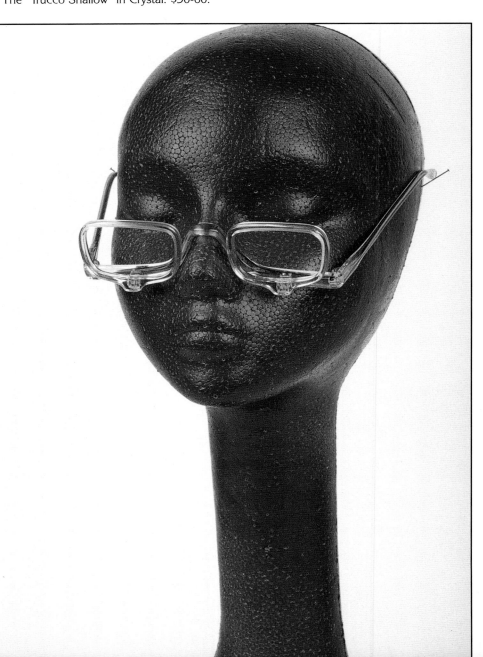

Hey! Can't you read the instructions? Only one side down at a time!

What big eyes you have! The "Trucco Deep" in Crystal. $50-60.

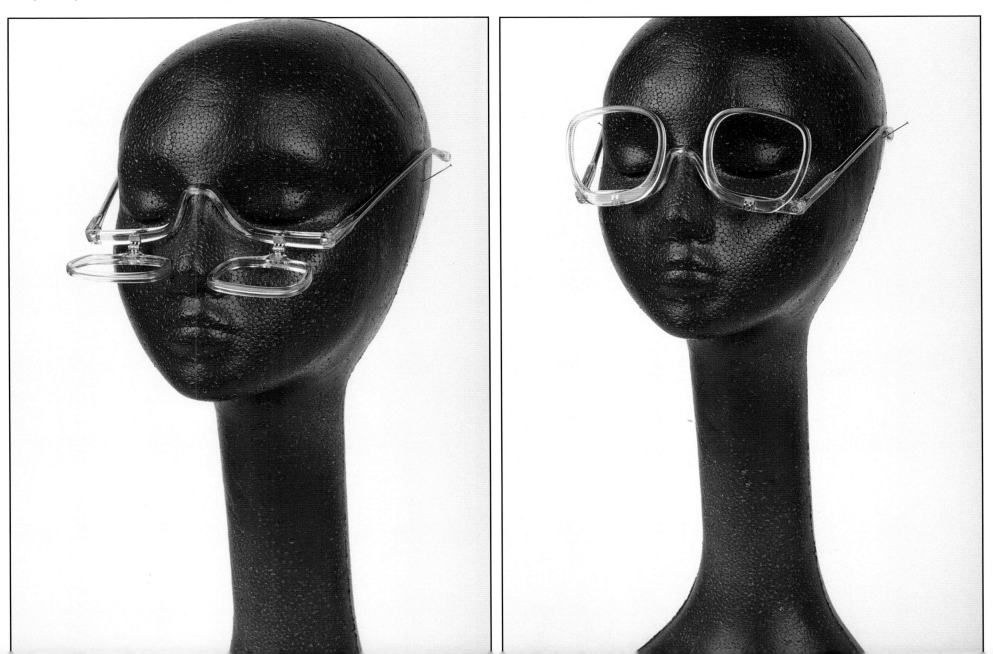

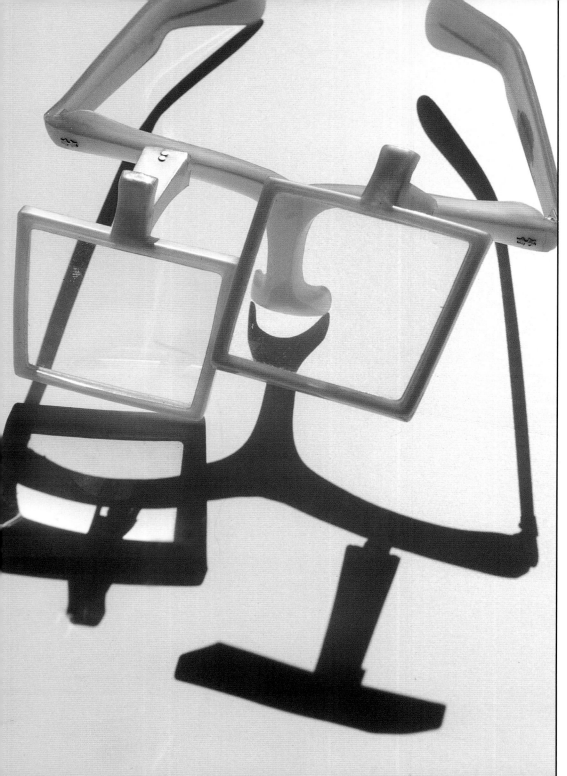

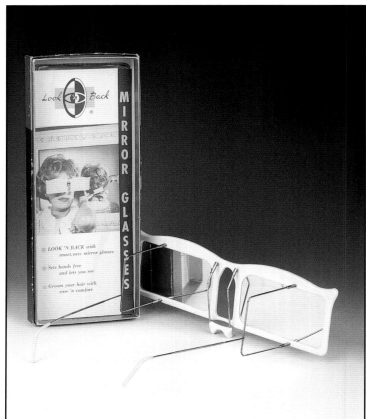

Wish you had eyes in the back of your head? Try these: Merco Manufacturing's "Look Back Mirror Glasses." "Sets hands free and lets you see!" $70-80.

Make-up specs in pale pink. $50-60.

Opposite page:
"I only wear them occasionally." If that's your line, folding glasses help keep your secret (for awhile, at least!). *Clockwise, from bottom left:* folding lorgnette, $70-80; men's folding tortoiseshell, $60-70; folding pink-and-rhinestone cat-eyes, $110-120; round dark amber and rhinestone, $110-120.

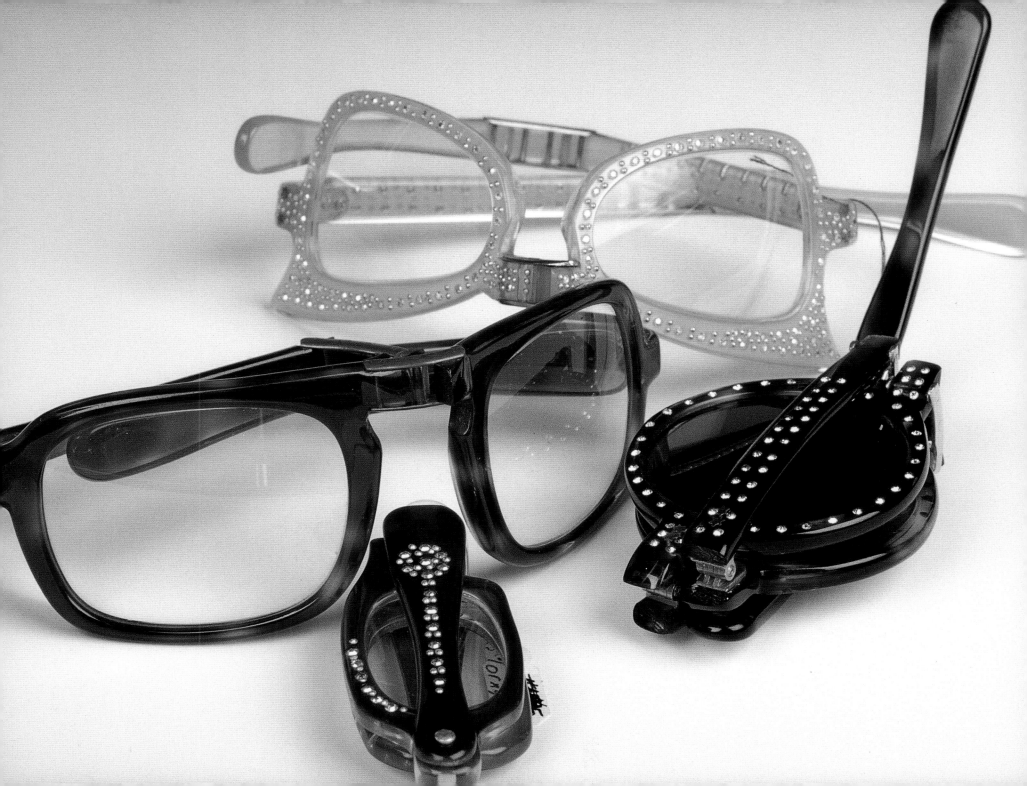

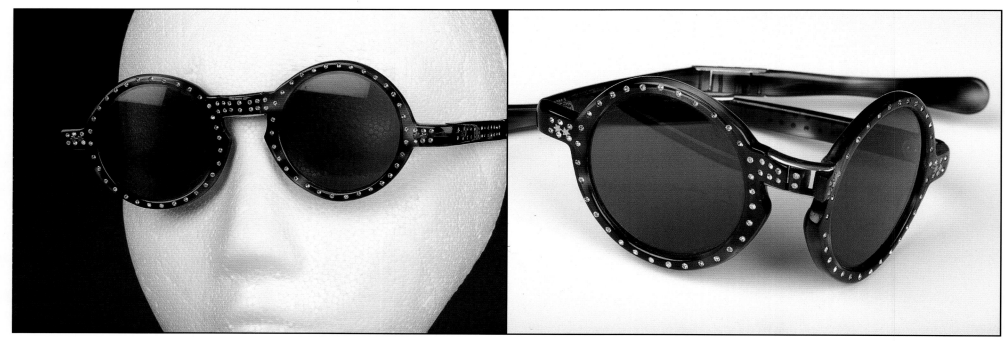

Detail, round dark amber foldups.

The same, folded.

A predecessor of modern folding glasses, was the folding oxford. It's shown here in a 1928 Bobrow Optical ad. The oxford was an adaptation of the French pince-nez, with spring action holding it in place.

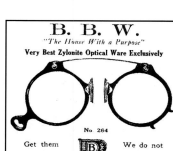

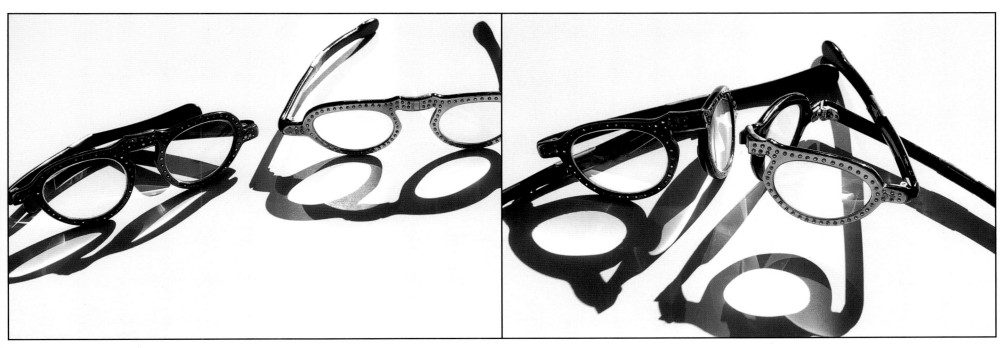

Dating from the 1930s and '40s, foldables from Paris. $175-200 each.

The foldables, folded.

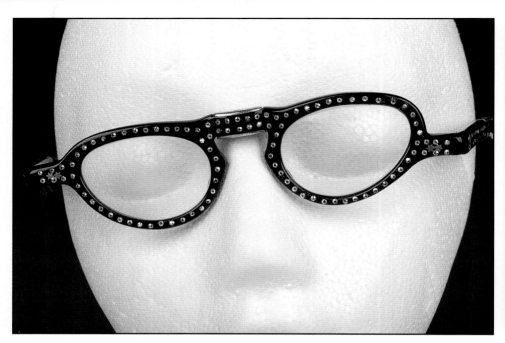

Black cat-eye foldups, with rhinestone outline. $110-120.

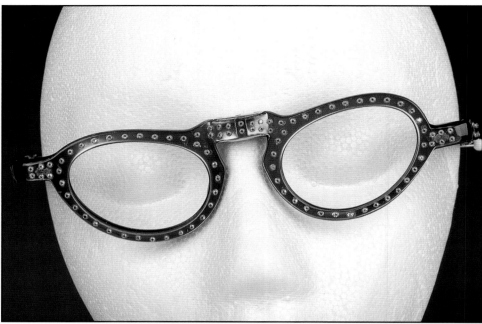

Folding cat-eyes in gold. $110-120.

Nicely tucked for traveling.

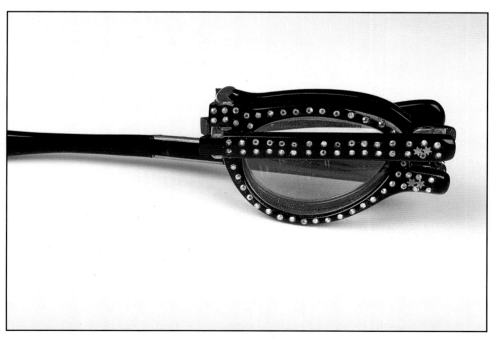

Opposite page:
Four pairs of French 1940s foldables. $150-175.

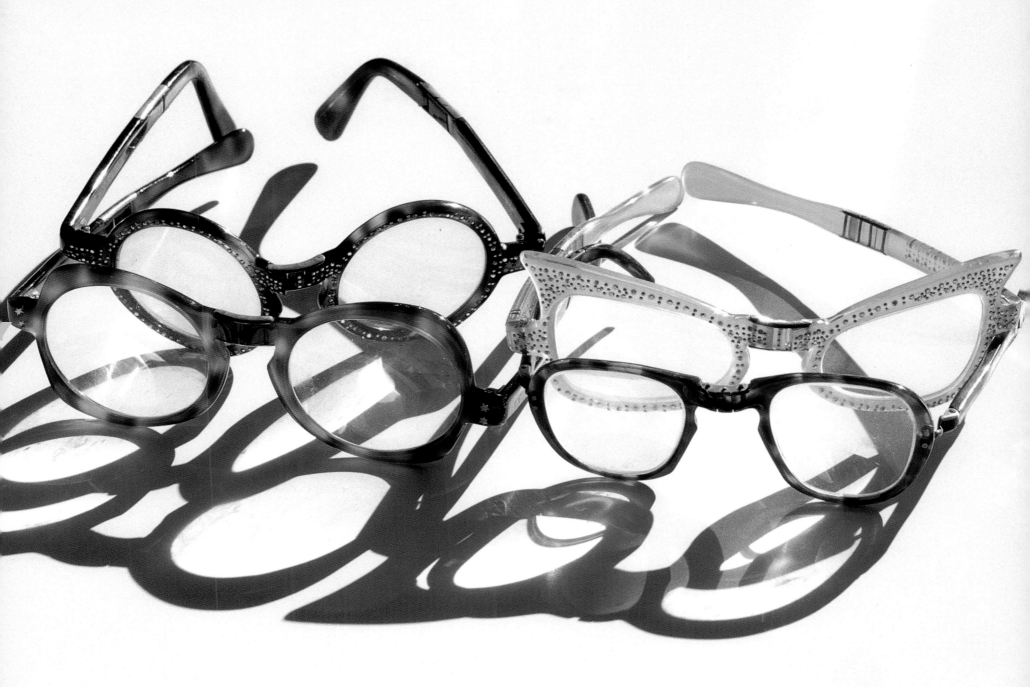

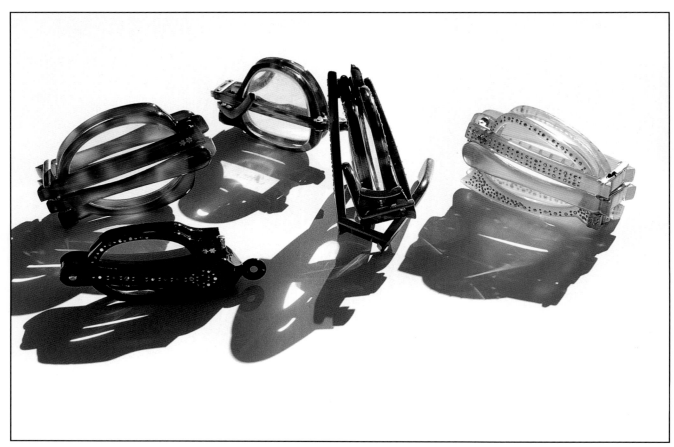

The four folded (plus one lorgnette!)

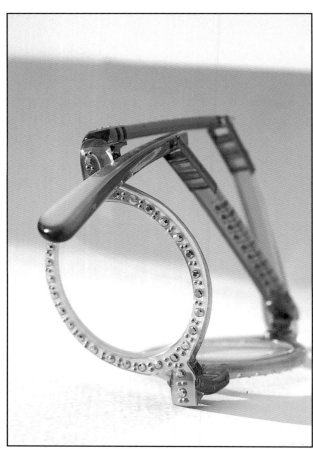

If you have to wear them, you might as well look good. Blue and silvery-grey foldups, ornamental enough for any optical occasion. $175-200.

Chapter 5:

"EYE-YI-YI!"

Novelty Eyewear, Accessories, & Display Ideas

First comic: "What did one pair of eyeglasses say to the other pair of eyeglasses?"
Second comic: "I don't know. What did one pair of eyeglasses say to the other pair of eyeglasses?"
First comic: "Must you make a spectacle of yourself?"
—Old vaudeville joke

Some mid-century eyewear does make a spectacle of itself, simply because it defies categorization. It may perform a unique function. It may stand alone, representative of a specific moment in time. It may be all that remains of a short-lived design idea...or it may have been created "just for fun."

Shown here are some of each: unique function frames, such as headband and radio glasses; time-specific ones, such as granny and earring glasses; short-lived design ideas like the "bandoleer". . . plus "eyelash glasses," "feather glasses," and others "just for fun."

Also included are spectacle cases, stands, chains, and other accessories intended to make life easier for the absentminded. And, there are several novel display ideas from eyewear collectors with plenty to display. There's an elegant presentation of glasses once owned by the Duchess of Windsor, a whimsical wire mannequin covered with novelty glasses, even frisky, vision-enhanced fish, and a perky poodle. One thing's for certain: when it comes to '50s and '60s novelty eyewear, you won't believe your eyes!

Unique In Function

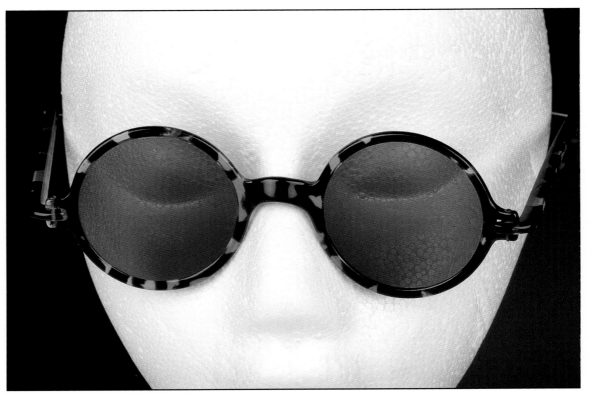

Like "looking at the world through rose-colored glasses?" These should help. Original rose-colored lenses in tortoiseshell frames. $70-80.

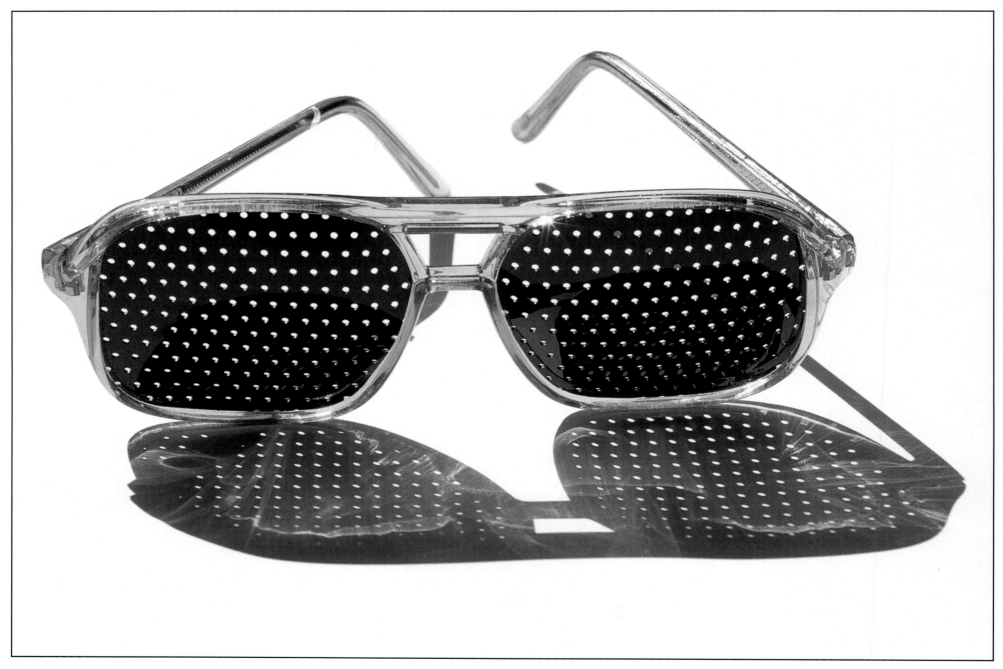

To your health! "Dr. Scholl's Health Glasses," designed to exercise flabby eye muscles, will have you seeing spots! $25-35.

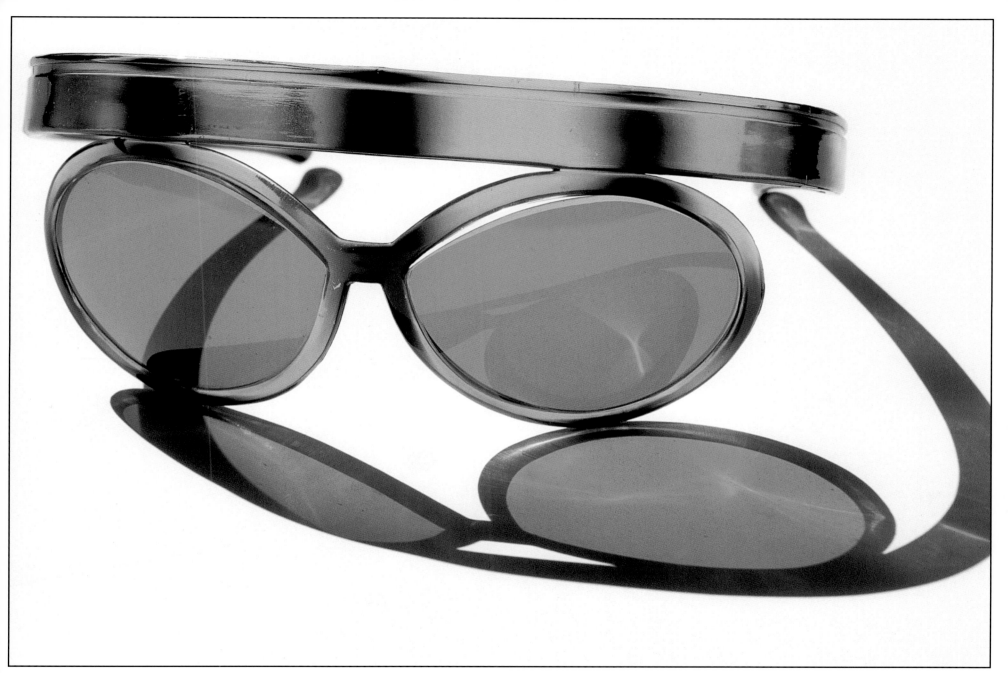

Save your ears for earrings. "Headband glasses" replace the usual temples with a tortoiseshell band. $250-275.

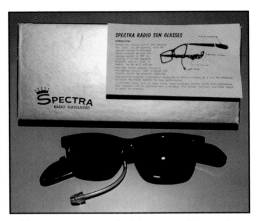

Never again miss the big game: Spectra's "radio sun glasses" keep you tuned in and turned on. $50-60.

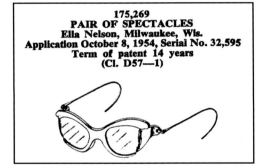

175,269
PAIR OF SPECTACLES
Ella Nelson, Milwaukee, Wis.
Application October 8, 1954, Serial No. 32,595
Term of patent 14 years
(Cl. D57—1)

Everybody wants into the act: Ella Nelson's 1955 patent for a "Pair Of Spectacles." Stylish, no—but they definitely won't slip off!

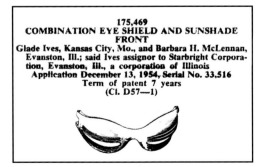

175,469
COMBINATION EYE SHIELD AND SUNSHADE FRONT
Glade Ives, Kansas City, Mo., and Barbara H. McLennan, Evanston, Ill.; said Ives assignor to Starbright Corporation, Evanston, Ill., a corporation of Illinois
Application December 13, 1954, Serial No. 33,516
Term of patent 7 years
(Cl. D57—1)

Wear it on the beach or wear it to bed. 1955 patent granted to the Starbright Corporation for a "Combination Eye Shield and Sunshade Front."

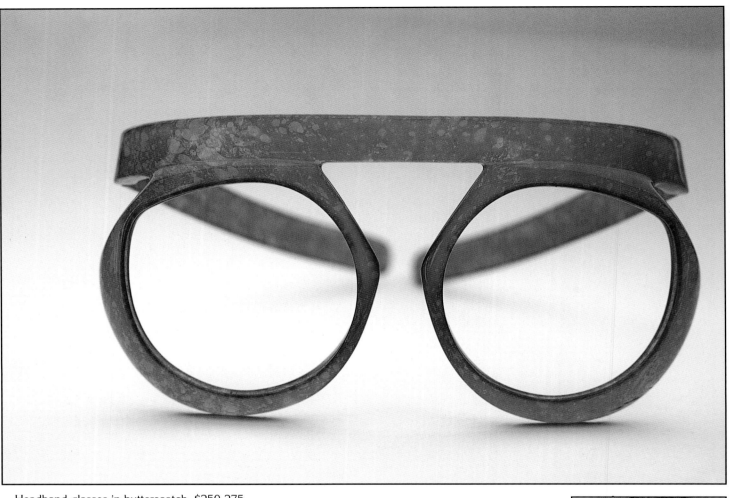

Headband glasses in butterscotch. $250-275.

The original "granny glasses!" This 1969 ad for "The Outasight Co." in *Seventeen* magazine offered original metal frames from the late 1800's. "Your optician puts in your prescription or plain or sun lenses." At the time, just $7.85.

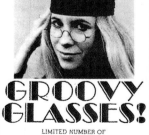

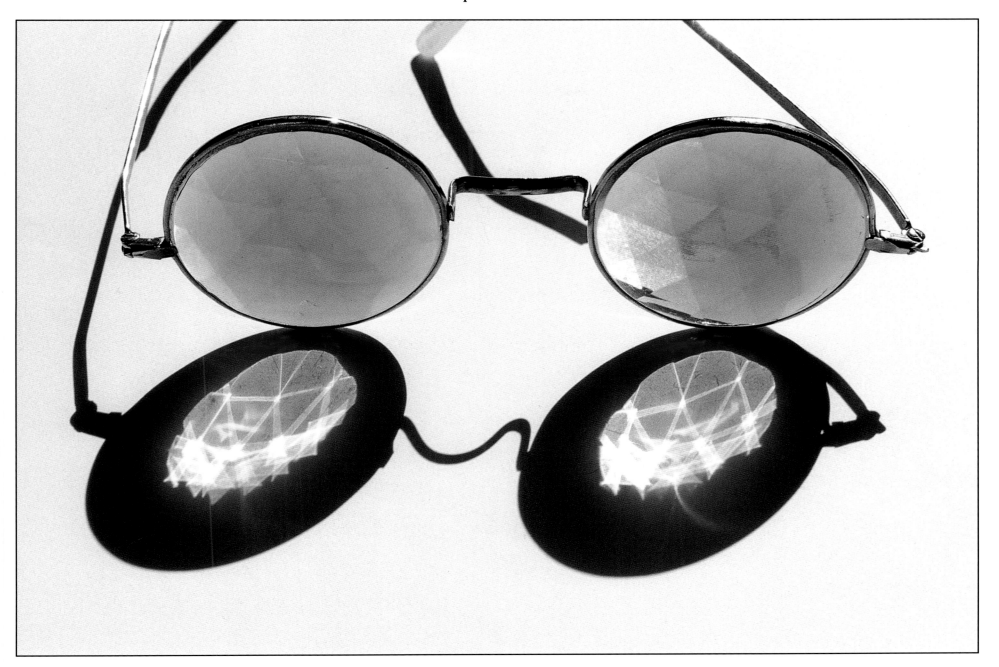

Groovy, baby! Faceted circular "hippie" (or "granny") glasses from the 1960s. The tinted prismatic lenses provide a rosy view of life. $60-75.

Totally wild! 1960s earring glasses in psyche-
delic black-and-white check. $120-160.

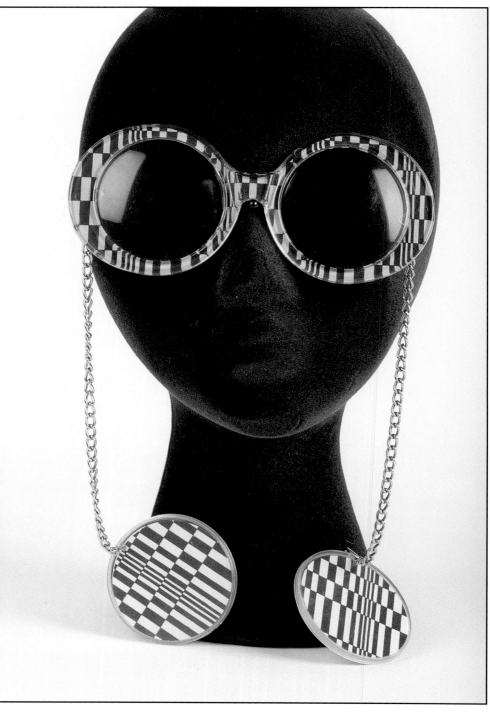

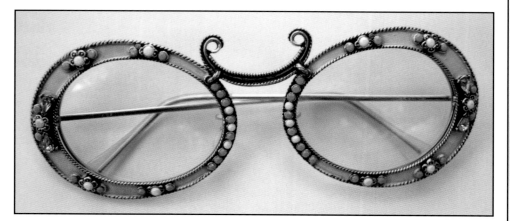

Christian Dior elegantly embraced the "granny glasses" style with these circular gold
metal frames, enhanced by a cloisonné-like border of blue enamel, rhinestones, and faux
pearls. $150-200.

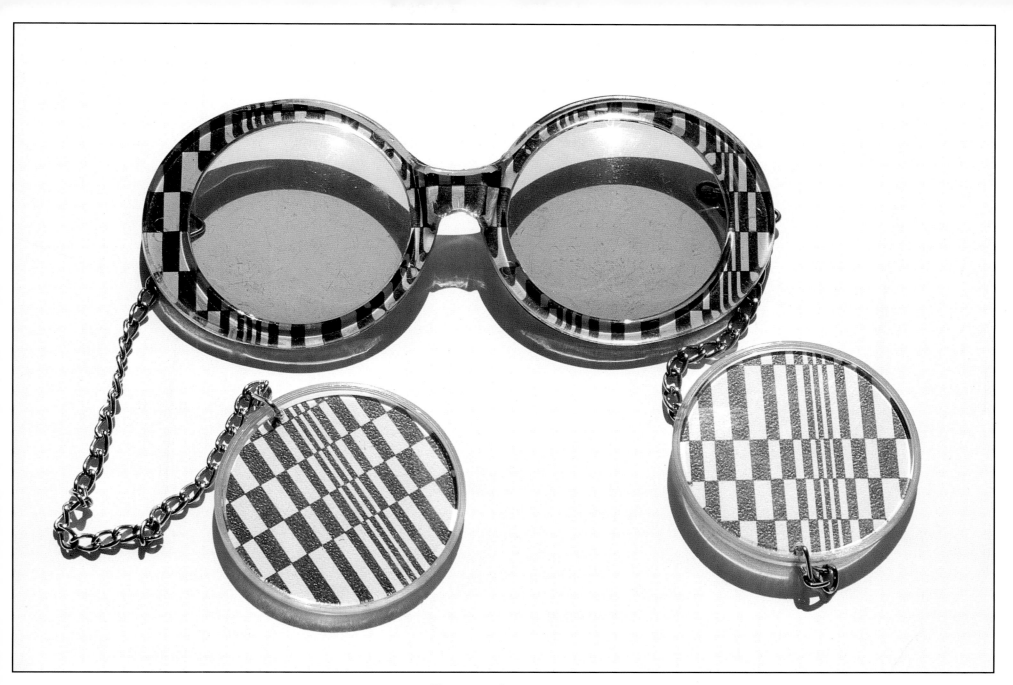

The earring glasses, at rest.

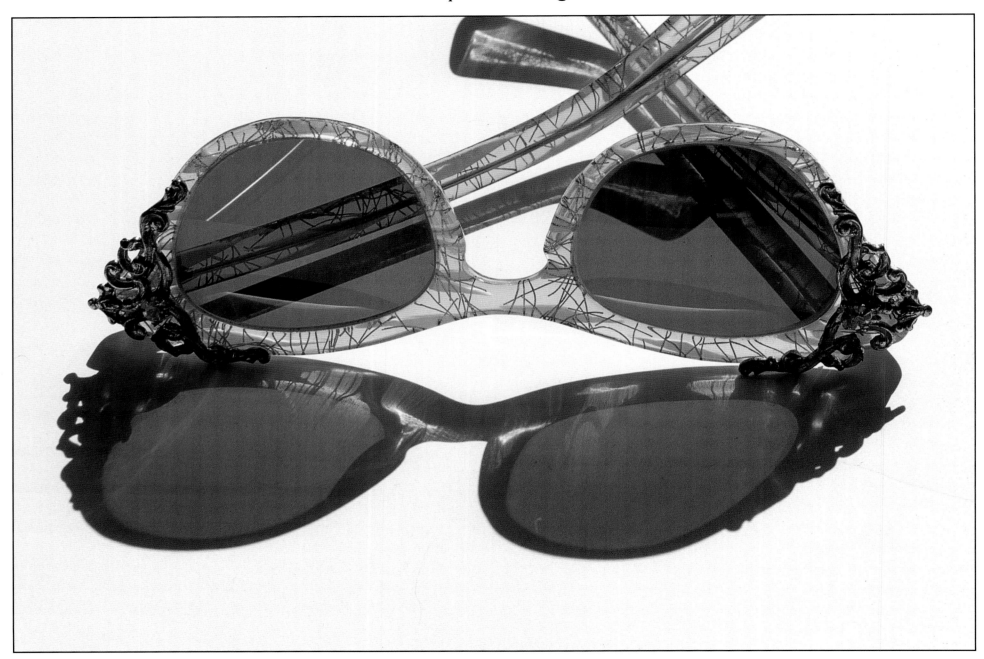

Almost Schiaparelli. Designer knock-offs provided celebrity style at a fraction of the cost. These gold string confetti frames feature Schiaparelli-like decorations at brow edge. $110-125.

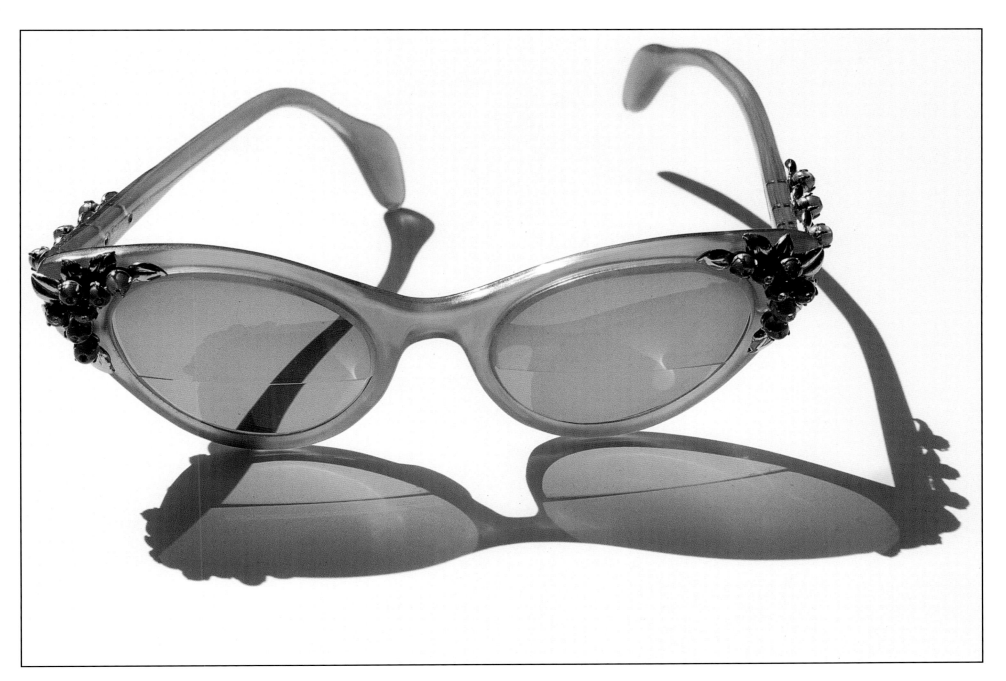

The real thing: clear yellow-gold Schiaparelli, with fruit clusters at brow and temple. $230-250.

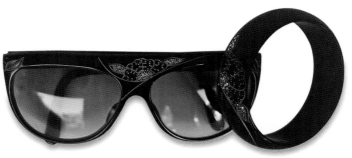

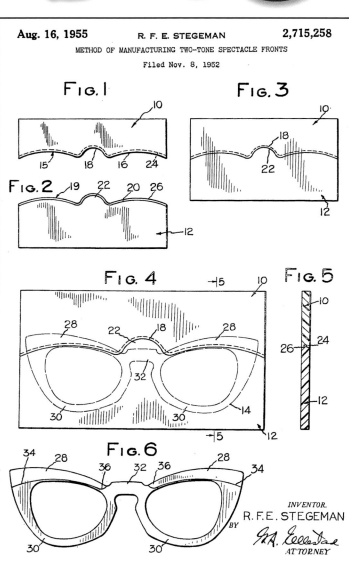

Aug. 16, 1955   R. F. E. STEGEMAN   2,715,258

METHOD OF MANUFACTURING TWO-TONE SPECTACLE FRONTS

Filed Nov. 8, 1952

FIG. 1

FIG. 3

FIG. 2

FIG. 4

FIG. 5

FIG. 6

INVENTOR.
R. F. E. STEGEMAN
BY
G.A. Gilletal
ATTORNEY

MAY Metal Frames

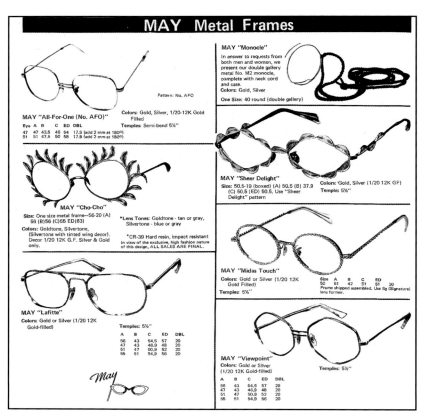

MAY "All-For-One (No. AFO)"

Eye	A	B	C	ED	DBL	
47	47	43.5	46	54	17.5	(add 2 mm at 180°)
51	51	47.5	50	58	17.5	(add 2 mm at 180°)

Pattern: No. AFO

Colors: Gold, Silver, 1/20-12K Gold Filled
Temples: Semi-bend 5½"

MAY "Monocle"

In answer to requests from both men and women, we present our double gallery metal No. M2 monocle, complete with neck cord and case.

Colors: Gold, Silver

One Size: 40 round (double gallery)

MAY "Cho-Cho"

Size: One size metal frame—56-20 (A) 56 (B)56 (C)55 ED(63)
Colors: Goldtone, Silvertone, (Silvertone with tinted wing decor). Decor 1/20 12K G.F. Silver & Gold only.

*Lens Tones: Goldtone - tan or gray, Silvertone - blue or gray

*CR-39 Hard resin, impact resistant in view of the exclusive, high fashion nature of this design, ALL SALES ARE FINAL.

MAY "Sheer Delight"

Size: 50.5-19 (boxed) (A) 50.5 (B) 37.9 (C) 50.5 (ED) 50.5. Use "Sheer Delight" pattern

Colors: Gold, Silver (1/20 12K GF)
Temple: 5½"

MAY "Lafitte"

Colors: Gold or Silver (1/20 12K Gold-filled)

A	B	C	ED	DBL
56	43	54.5	57	20
47	43	46.9	48	20
51	47	60.9	52	20
55	51	54.9	56	20

MAY "Midas Touch"

Colors: Gold or Silver (1/20 12K Gold Filled)
Temples: 5½"

Size	A	B	C	ED
50	51	42	51	51	20

Frame shipped assembled. Use Sg (Signature) lens former.

MAY "Viewpoint"

Colors: Gold or Silver (1/20 12K Gold-filled)

A	B	C	ED	DBL
56	43	54.5	57	20
47	43	46.9	48	20
51	47	50.9	52	20
55	51	54.9	56	20

Temples: 5½"

May

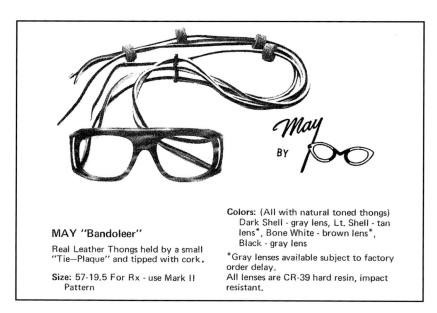

MAY "Bandoleer"

Real Leather Thongs held by a small "Tie—Plaque" and tipped with cork.

Size: 57-19.5 For Rx - use Mark II Pattern

Colors: (All with natural toned thongs) Dark Shell - gray lens, Lt. Shell - tan lens*, Bone White - brown lens*, Black - gray lens

*Gray lenses available subject to factory order delay.
All lenses are CR-39 hard resin, impact resistant.

May BY

Top left: Matched set: glasses and bracelet by Stendahl, for the well-coordinated ensemble. $150-200.

Bottom left: What's your best color? Why decide? Go for more than one, with "two-tone spectacle fronts." Raymond Stegeman's 1955 patent description states that "the upper brow portions are formed of one color material, the bridge and remaining rim portions formed of material of a different color." The presumably colorful finished product was manufactured by Bausch & Lomb.

Top right: Frame possibilities are endless. Some 1972 May selections include the leafy "Cho-Cho," the twisting "Sheer Delight," and that old standby—the "Monocle!"

Bottom right: Mrs. Zorro would love these. Also by May, the "Bandoleer," with temples replaced by "real leather thongs held by a small 'tie-plaque' and tipped with cork." Olé!

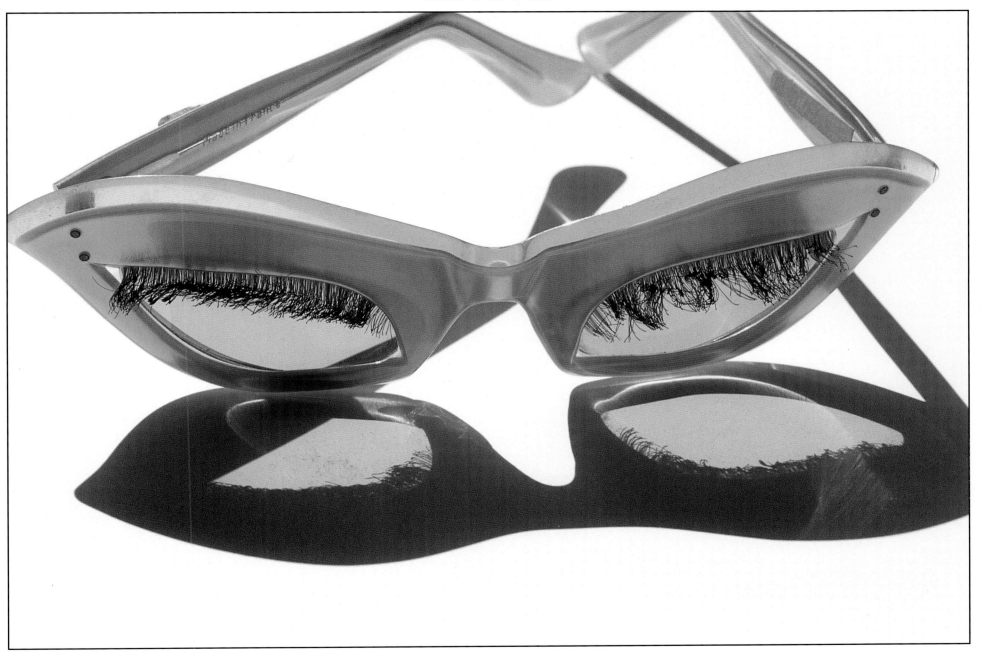

Longing for long, luxuriant eyelashes? Solve the problem with "eyelash glasses." Definitely on the fringe! $350-375.

Just for kids (or those with small heads):
Japanese "spaceman" sun glasses in
virulent day-glo orange. $120-130.

Making beautiful music: highbrows in the form of musical
notes. $375-400.

122

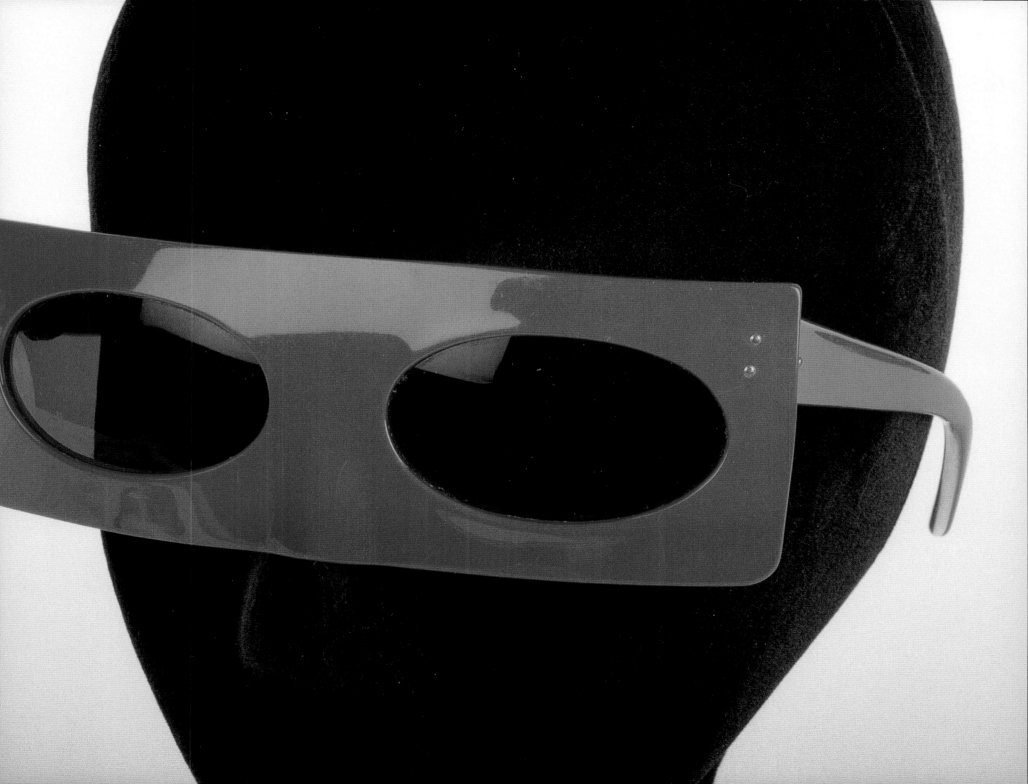

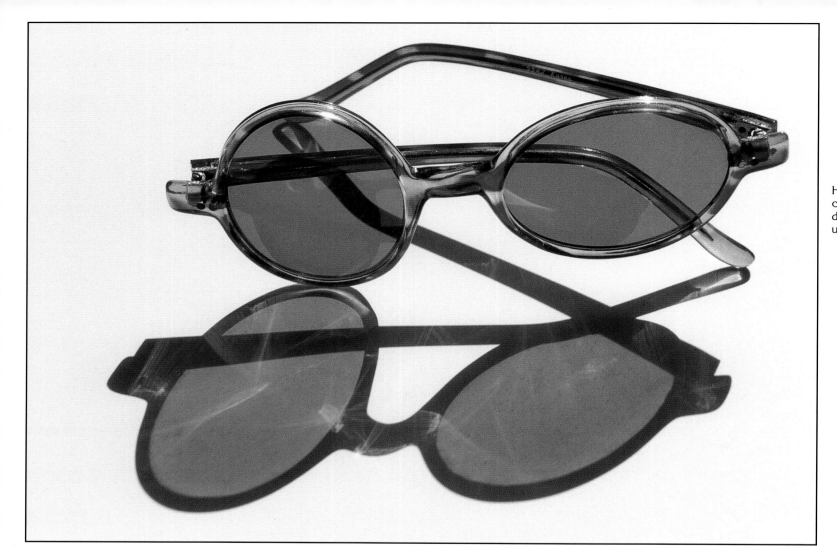

Here's an eye-popper: one lens circular, the other oval, for those days when you just can't make up your mind! $35-50.

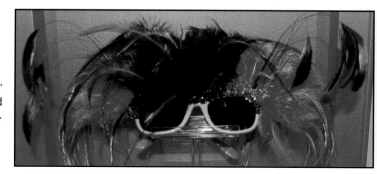

Feathered friend: "feather glasses" do double duty as sun glasses and hair decoration. $150-200.

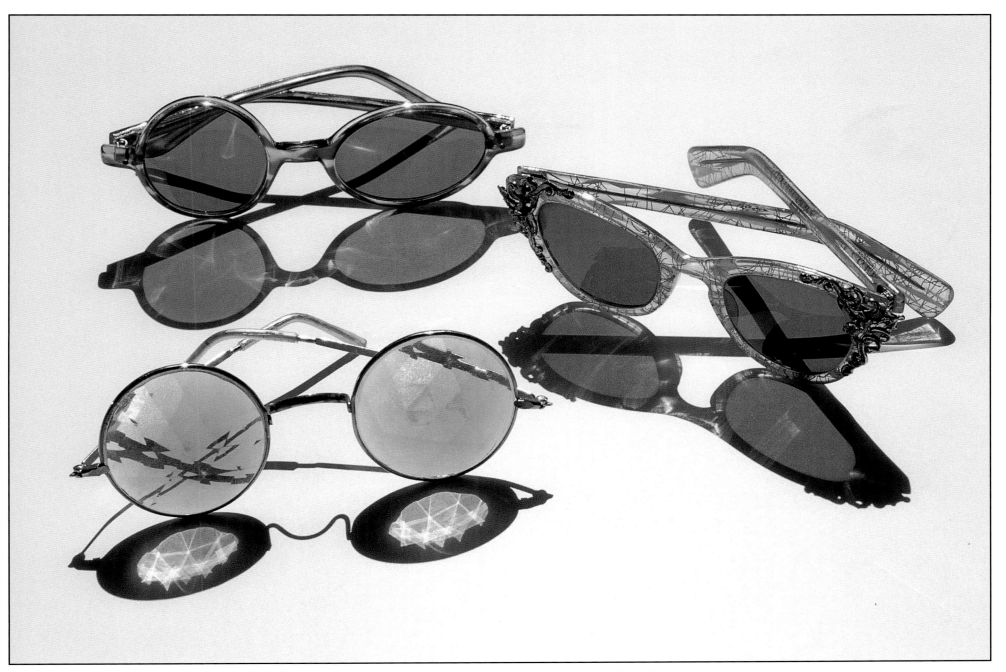

Ready for any occasion: granny glasses, mismatched lenses, and faux Schiaparelli.

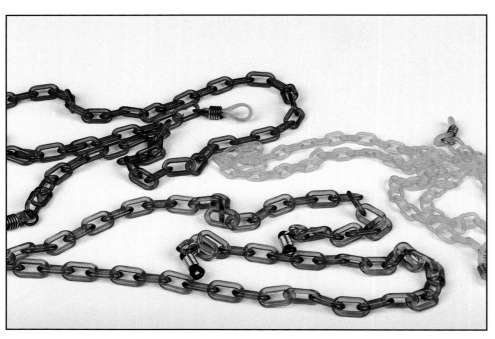

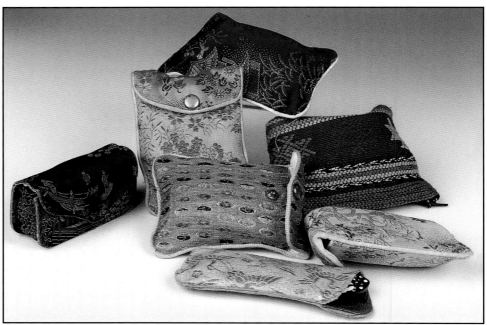

2,708,025
SPECTACLE CASES AND METHOD OF MAKING SAME
Charles A. Baratelli, Southbridge, Mass., assignor to American Optical Company, Southbridge, Mass., a voluntary association of Massachusetts
Application March 24, 1953, Serial No. 344,294
5 Claims. (Cl. 206—5)

1. A spectacle case embodying a main pocket portion and an integral flap portion formed of flexible sheet material, said main pocket portion comprising two sections divided by a scored line and having identical end edge contours, said sections being folded along said scored line to provide bottom marginal portions and said end edge contours in superimposed relation with each other, said bottom marginal portions and adjacent end edge contours of said two sections being secured together by a line of stitching, a cuplike liner of injection molded plastic material having spaced front and rear wall portions integrally joined with each other along the sides and bottom thereof by portions curving in arcs of relatively short radii to retain said front and rear wall portions in said spaced relation with each other, said liner being positioned in said pocket portion and being shaped and dimensioned so as to have a relatively intimate fit with said pocket portion, said flap extending from the rear section of the pocket portion and foldable over the front section thereof, the respective front section of said pocket portion and front wall of said liner each having an aligned opening therein, snap fastener means having a portion extending through said aligned openings and secured therein, said integral flap portion having a separate depending tongue thereon, and snap fastener means connected with said tongue and being adapted to be detachably connected with the other snap fastener means carried by the front section of the pocket portion and front wall of the liner to secure the snap in place over said front section of the pocket portion.

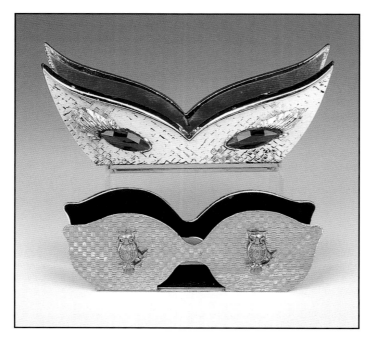

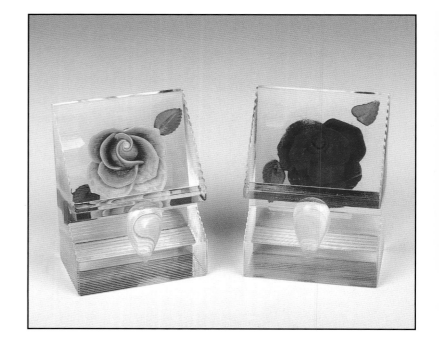

Made To Be Seen

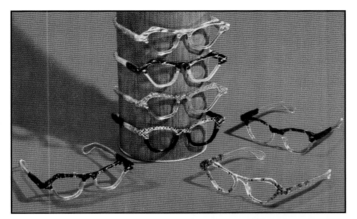

Showing it off: display ideas from Lumar, circa mid-1950s.

Opposite page:

Top left: To keep things from going astray: festive eyeglass chains in amber, gray, and yellow. $10-15 each.

Top right: An array of attractively-patterned eyeglass cases from the 1950s and '60s. Under $10 each.

Bottom left: "Spectacle Cases And Method Of Making Same," a 1955 patent design by Charles A. Baratelli for American Optical Company.

Bottom center: Here's looking at you, kid! These vintage eyeglass stands are an eyeful in themselves. $10-15 each.

Bottom right: Lucite eyeglass stands, just right for the boudoir, featuring back-carved floral designs. $15-20 each.

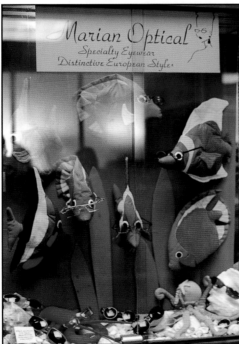

The original "wall-eyes?" Fish in glasses, an entertaining display from Marian Optical, St. John's, Newfoundland.

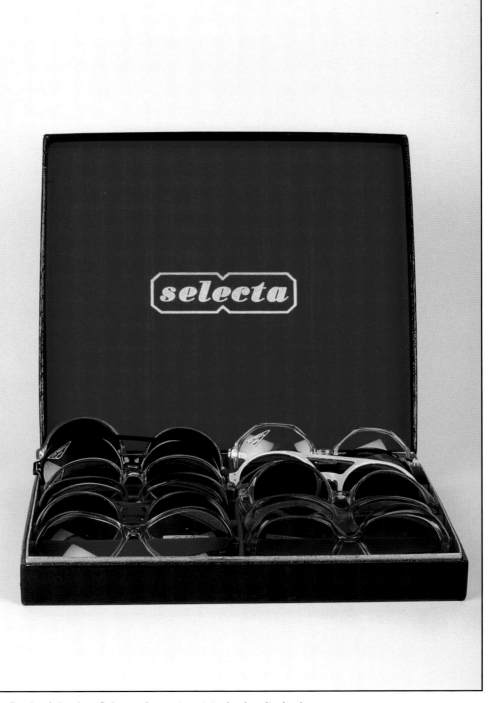

Catch of the day: Selecta glasses in original sales display box.

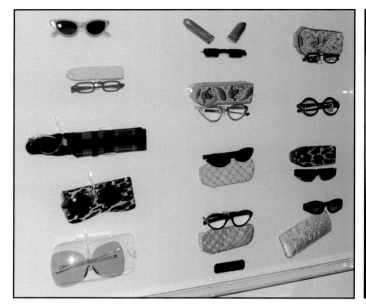

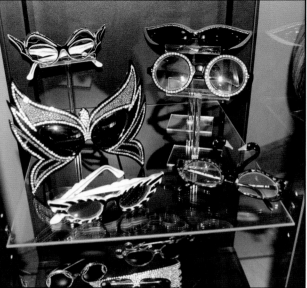

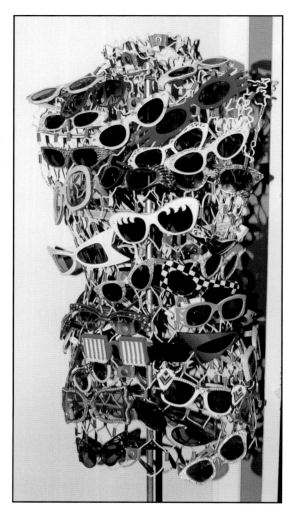

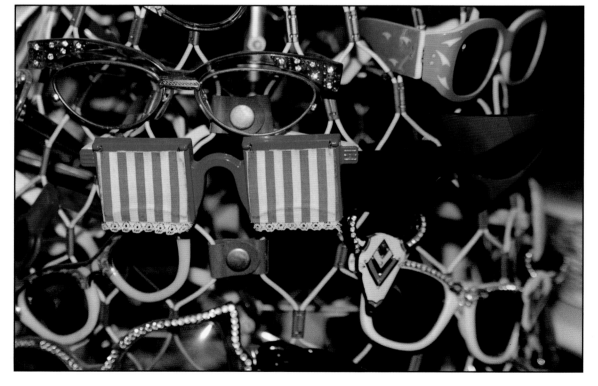

Top left: Lifestyles of the rich and famous: glasses from the estate of the Duchess of Windsor, now in the collection of Marilyn Cohen.

Top center: Glasses on glass: display ideas from the Marilyn Cohen Collection.

Top Right: Body of work: wire mannequin covered in novelty glasses from the Marilyn Cohen Collection.

Bottom: Marilyn Cohen novelty glasses, including, at center, a pair with striped awnings!

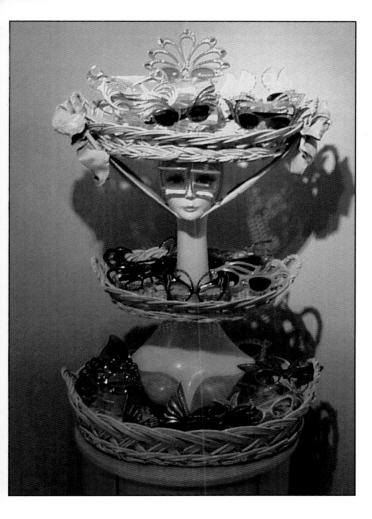

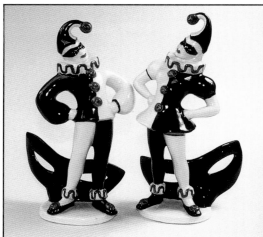

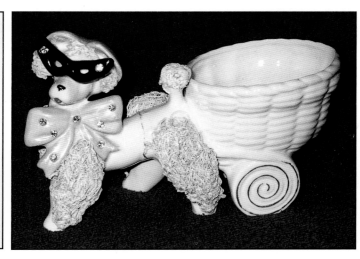

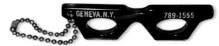

Top left: A mannequin head is festooned with wicker baskets, turning all eyes to glasses from the Ellen Foster Collection. The stand originally served as a department store display for lingerie.

Top center: Harlequins in harlequins. This "Harlequin Boy and Girl" wear the sort of masks that inspired the harlequin and cat-eye glasses of the 1950s. The enchanting figurines were designed by Betty Harrington for Ceramic Arts Studio.

Top right: Looking arf-lly good! "Glenda," a spaghetti art ware poodle of the mid-50s, swallows her pride and models black cat-eyes with rhinestone studs. During the 1950s, California and Japan-made poodles in eyewear were nifty knickknacks. They can still be found by today's determinedly "dogged" collector! $40-50.

Bottom: Keeping an eye on your keys: novelty eyeglass keychain from G.E. Waldron, Geneva, New York.

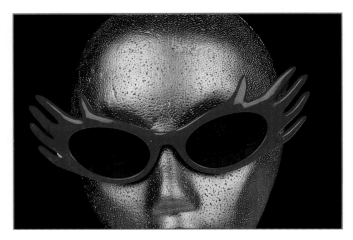

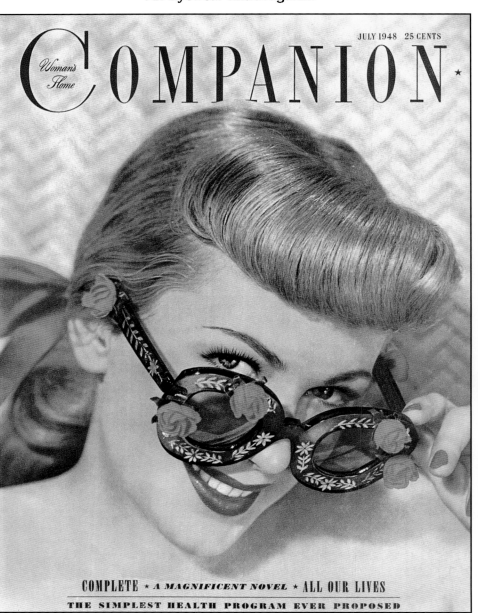

JULY 1948 25 CENTS

Woman's Home COMPANION ★

COMPLETE ★ *A MAGNIFICENT NOVEL* ★ ALL OUR LIVES
THE SIMPLEST HEALTH PROGRAM EVER PROPOSED

There is nothing very special about saving money; all it takes is money. Spending it is trickier: show us a woman who spends well—with wit, with wisdom, and with relish—and we'll show you a cloudless disposition, an unfurrowed brow, and a superior digestion; a monument, in fact, to savoir vivre.
—*Vogue*
April, 1962

The "woman who spends well," lauded by *Vogue* in a fashion layout of the early '60s, was, incidentally, doing all that spending while wearing glasses. And not just any glasses, either: these were extravagant, eye-filling, *expensive* glasses. The sort of glasses most *Vogue* readers would give their eye-teeth for. The sort of glasses shown here.

Set your sights on these: some of the most superbly theatrical eyewear designs of the 1950s and '60s. Heavenly highbrows. Beauteous butterflies. Splendiferous swans. Winged wonders. Each lovelier than the last. Each destined to turn its wearer into a vision of loveliness.

This spec-tacular glasswear gallery features many of the most desirable (and, inevitably, most expensive) creations in eyewear fashion. They represent the pinnacle. Considering the prices, in this case one pair *may* be enough...until the next one. So keep your eye on the prize; it's worth it. In the words of "Miss Specs," "of *course* men make passes at girls who wear glasses. It simply depends on the frame."

Sultry in sun glasses: *Vogue* cover girl of the 1940s.

More homespun: this *Woman's Home Companion* cover girl makes a run for the roses in flower-bedecked sun glasses. July, 1948.

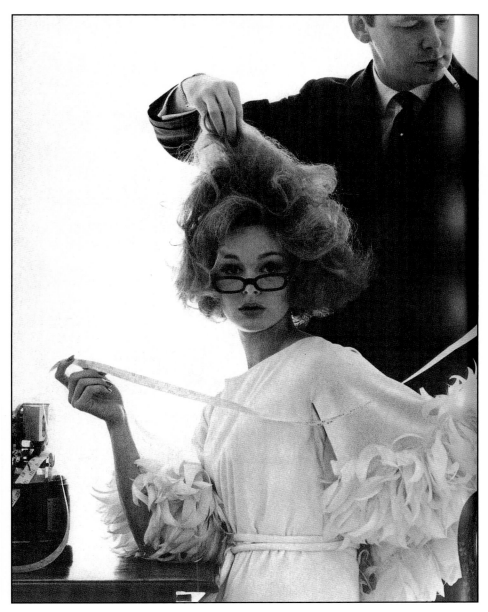

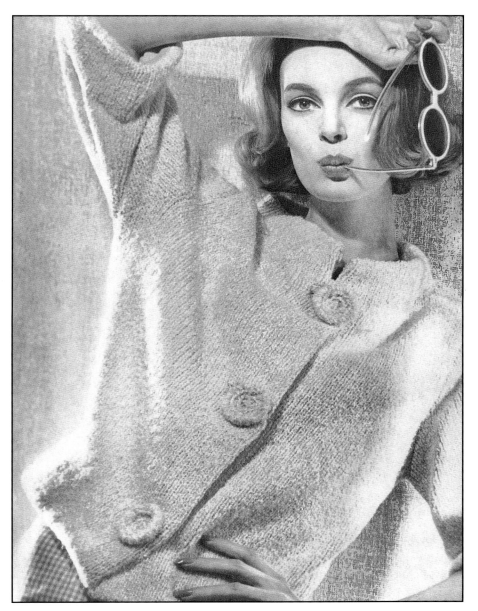

Such elaborate lives: *Vogue*'s 1962 "woman who spends well" ("of unguessable years and unfathomable millions") has it all. There's her "floor-length at-home dress by Christian Dior, of white silk crepe, wrapped, sashed, and up to its elbows in coq feathers." There's "Kenneth, the very best hairdresser that money can buy." There's her "very own ticker tape machine from Hammacher-Schlemmer." Oh, and there are her extravagantly oversized glasses, for that working-girl touch.

Glasses meant for posing: June, 1962 *Vogue* model with "sun glasses by May at Lugene."

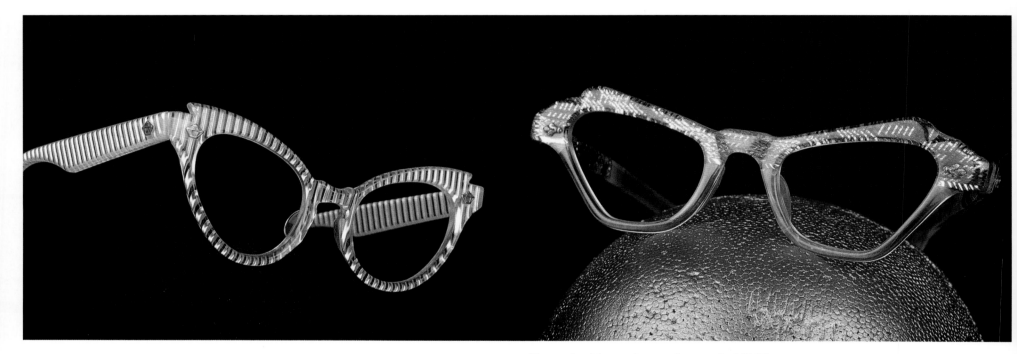

Simply splendid stripes: clear stripe frames by Lumar. $90-105.

Blue and gold meet for a perfect mesh. $60-70.

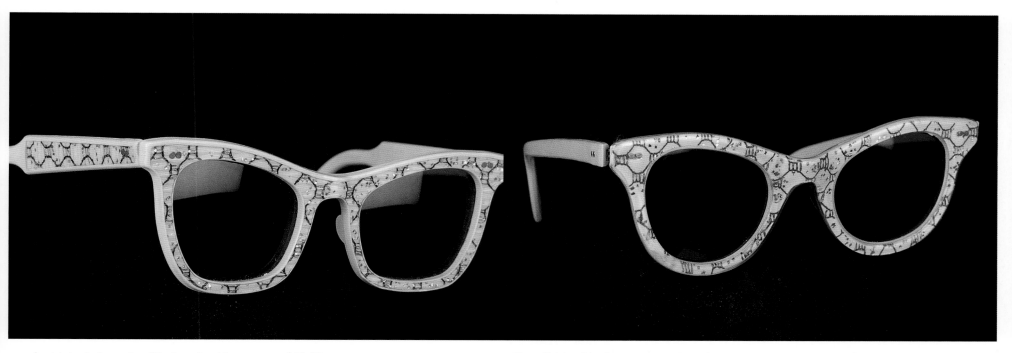

Lavish look, low price. Black and gold on cream, $40-50.

Beautiful (and budget-conscious): multi-color glitter on light blue. $50-60.

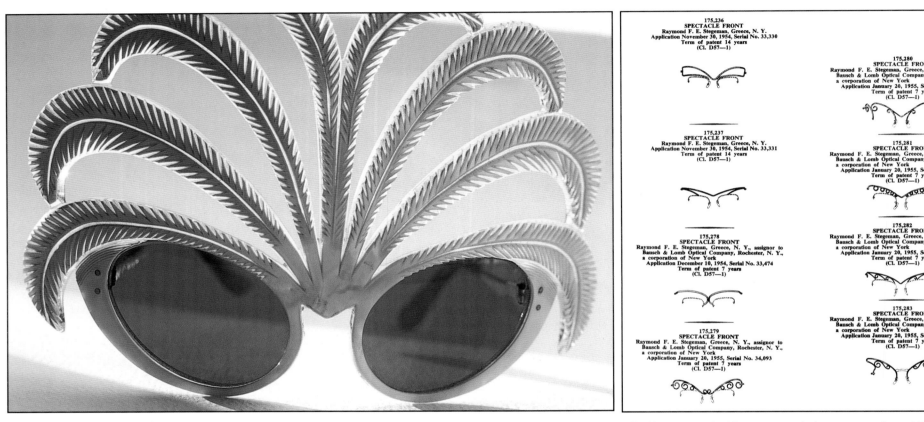

Opulent feathery palm highbrows in beige and cream. French, $1000-1200.

Builder-uppers: highbrow spectacle front patents from 1955.

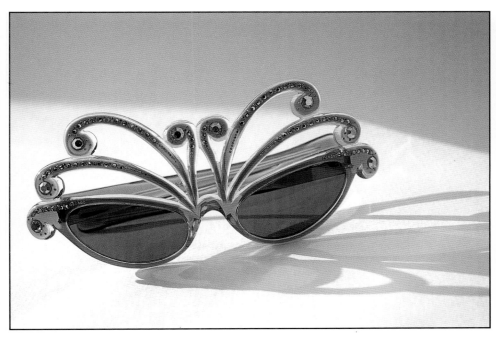

Entrancing smokey coffee antenna highbrows with aurora rhinestones. France, $375-400.

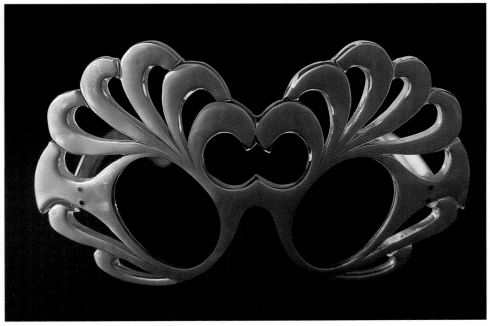

Pearl and clear rhinestone plumes. $600-650.

Fantasy black and rhinestone plumes on clear plastic. Frame France, $600-650.

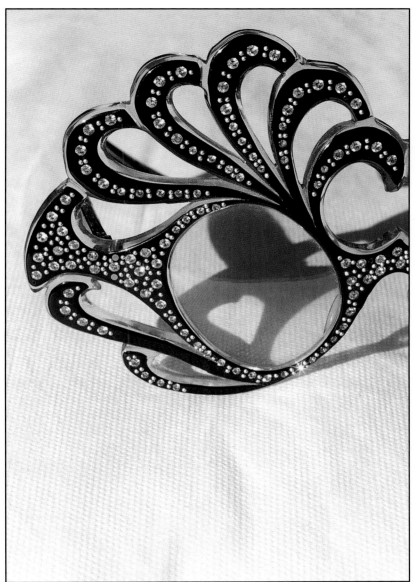

Plume detail.

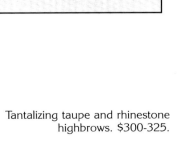

Tantalizing taupe and rhinestone
highbrows. $300-325.

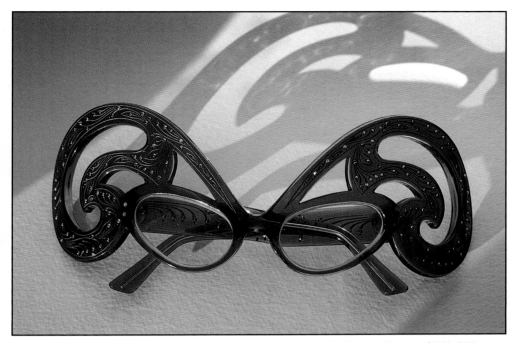

Captivating "ram horn" highbrows. Brown with rhinestones by Qualite France. $550-600.

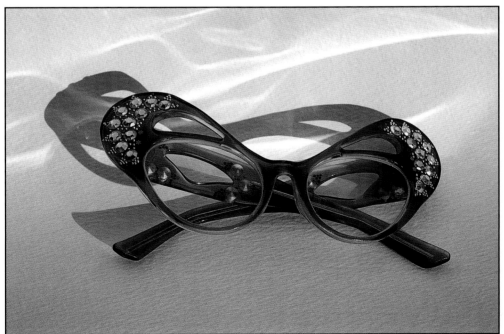

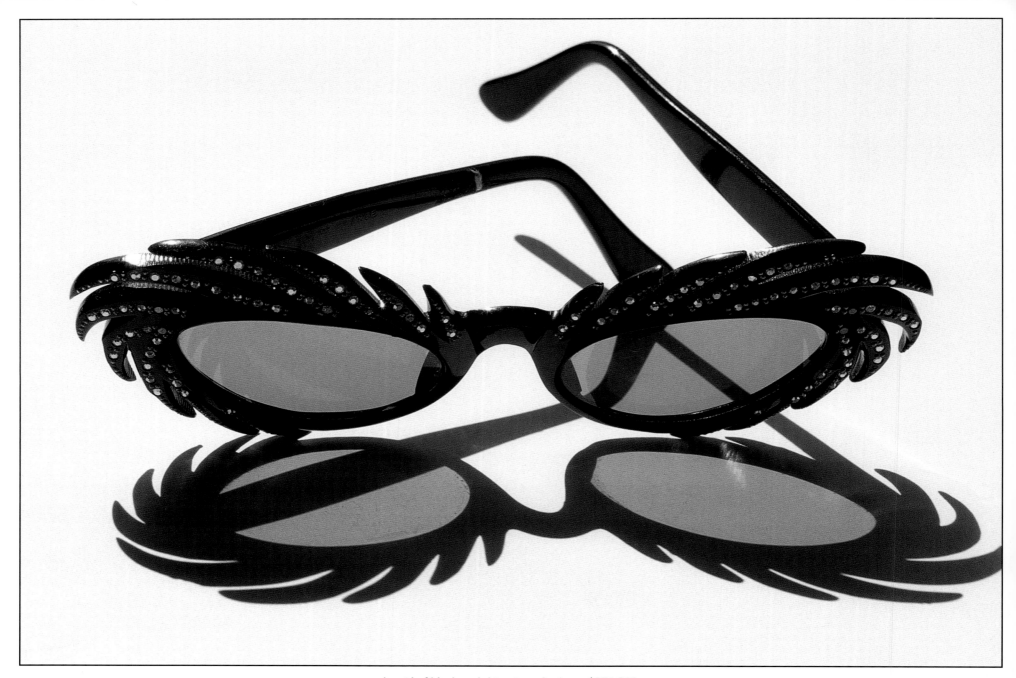

A swirl of black and rhinestone feathers. $275-300.

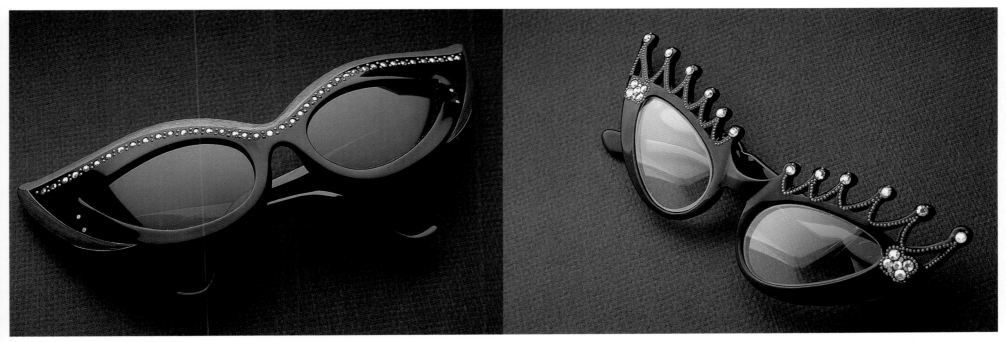

Glorious gold and black cat-eyes with aurora rhinestone band. French, $175-200.

Crowning glory: black crown brows with aurora rhinestone tips. French, $225-250.

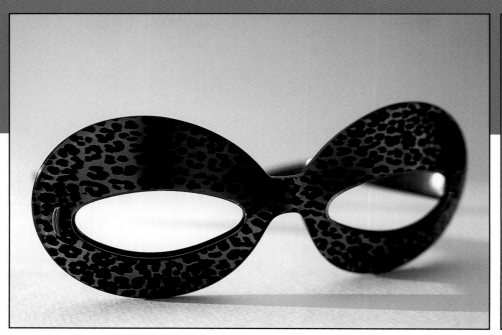

On the prowl: leopard-print slits, $250-275.

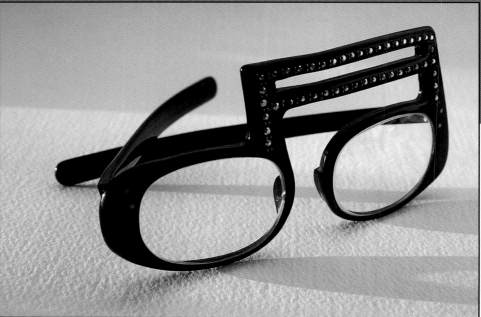

Hitting all the right notes: musical note highbrows in black with rhinestone accents. French, $375-400.

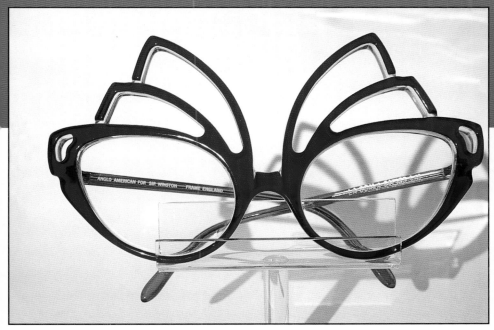

Seeing triple: red highbrows, with repeating brow shape. Marked "Anglo American for Sir Winston. Frame England." $375-400.

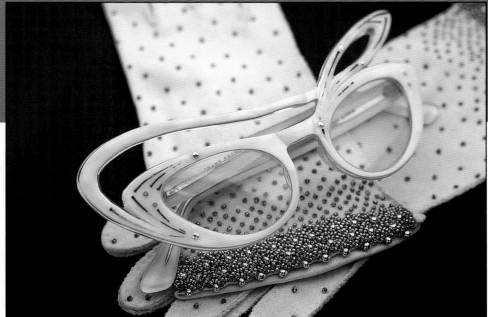

Luxuriant looped brow, in cream with silver studs. French, by Mona Lisa. $275-300.

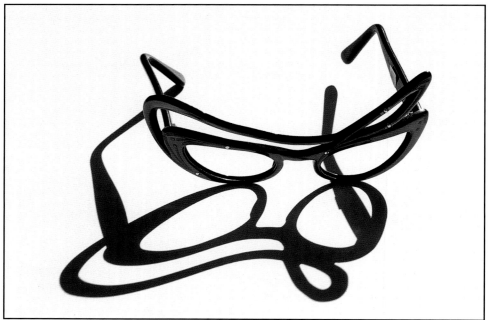

Looping the loop: the same, in brown with gold studs. $275-300.

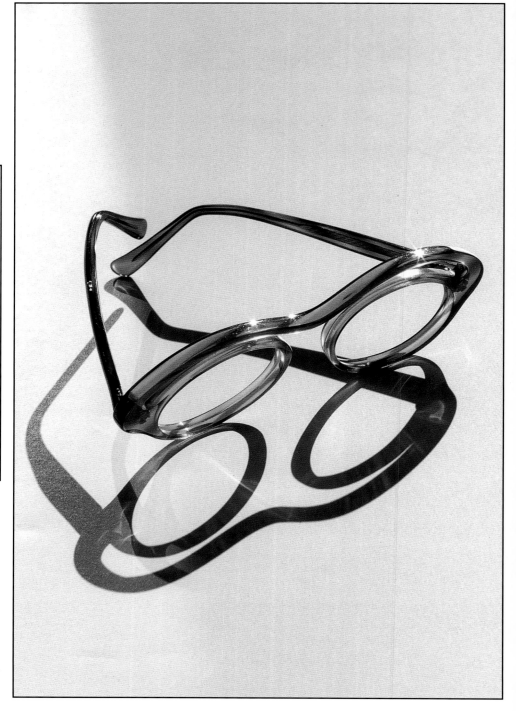

Still loopy: by Raphael, from 1930s Paris. $140-160.

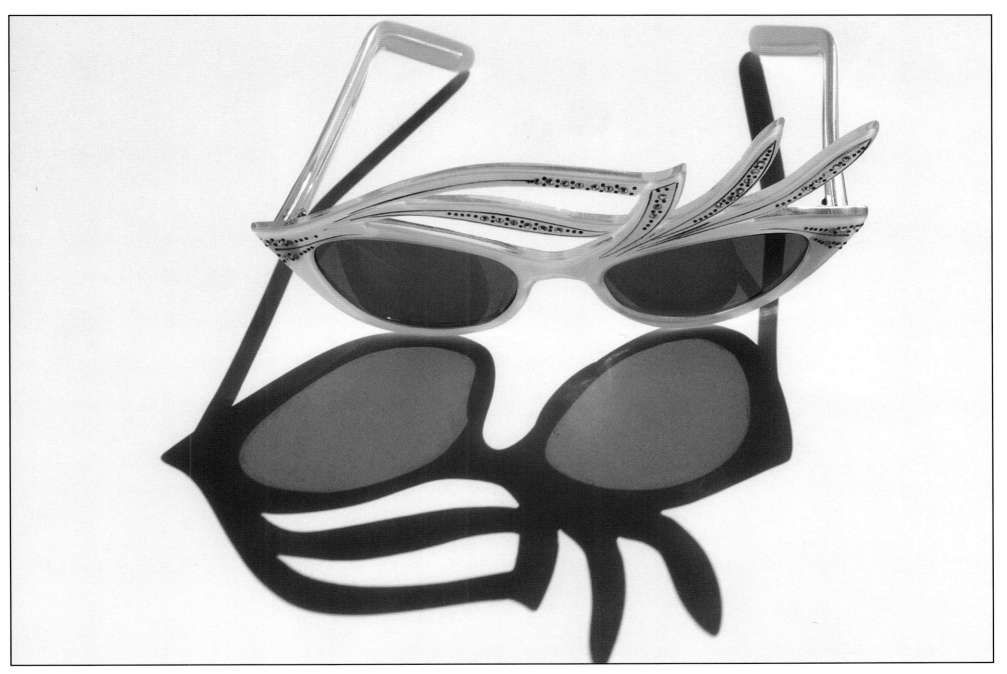

Mellow yellow with asymmetrical brow. $200-300.

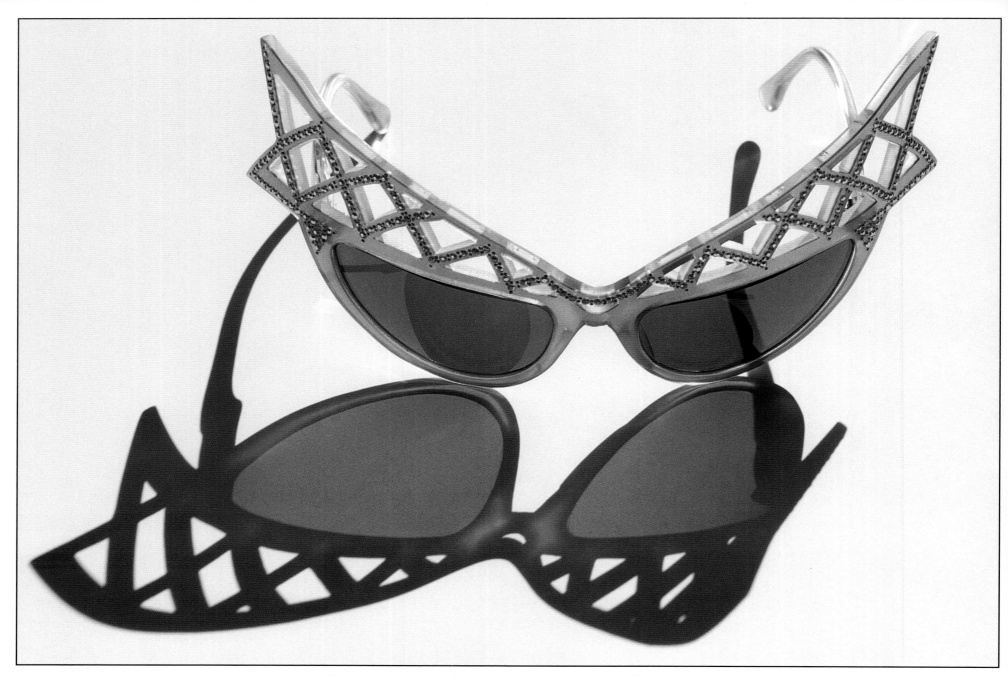

Passionate purple, with rhinestone crosshatching on brow. $300-400.

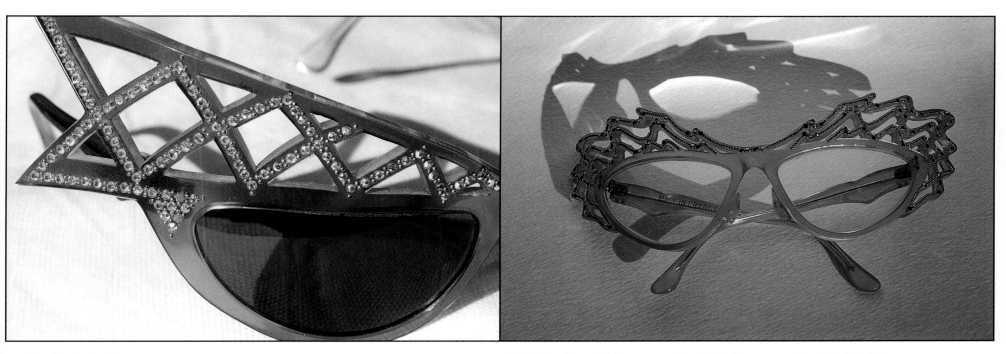

Crosshatch detail.

Rippled yellow-gold brows, garnished with rhinestones. French, $400-425.

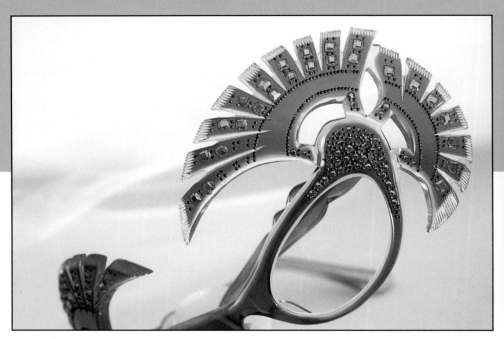

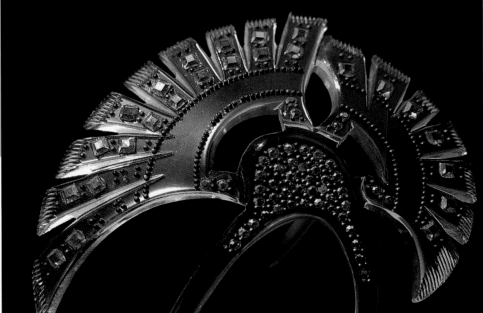

Fan-tastic! Magnificent brow edge fan shapes in purple, encrusted with rhinestones. $600-650.

Fan detail.

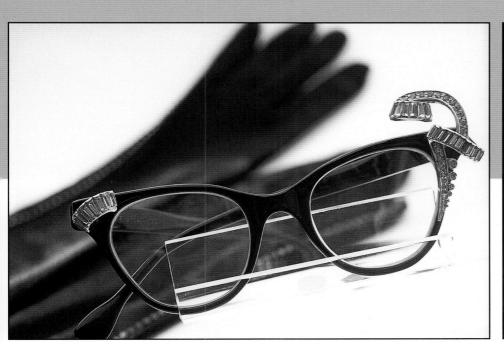

Romantic in rhinestones. Basic black, offset by lush rhinestone ornaments at brow edge. $275-300.

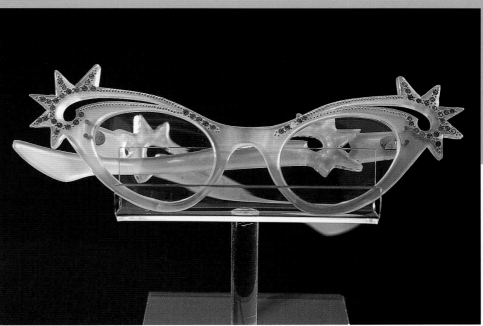

Seeing stars: pink plastic frames with rhinestone star shapes. $350-375.

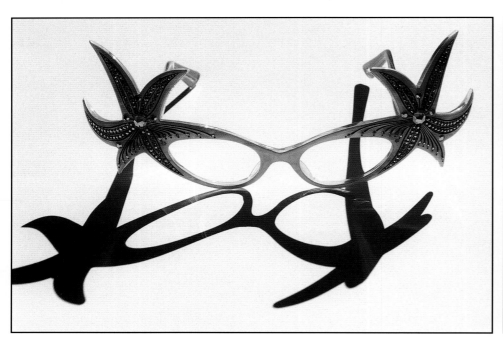

Sensational star-flowers with rhinestone centers and petals. $300-400.

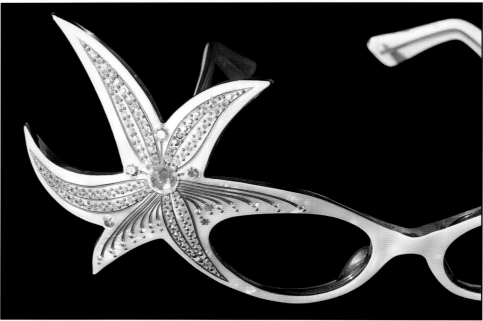

Star-flower detail.

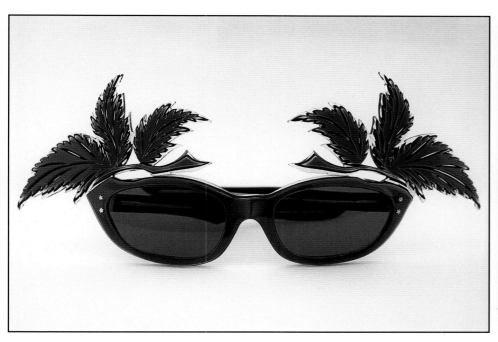

Branching out: smokey-brown leaves sprout from brow edges. French, $500-550.

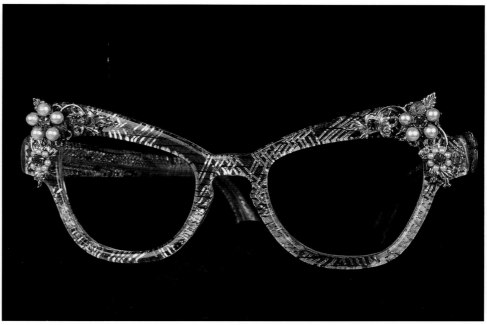

For a lustrous night: black-and-gold mesh, with pearl and blue rhinestone clusters at brow edge. $120-140.

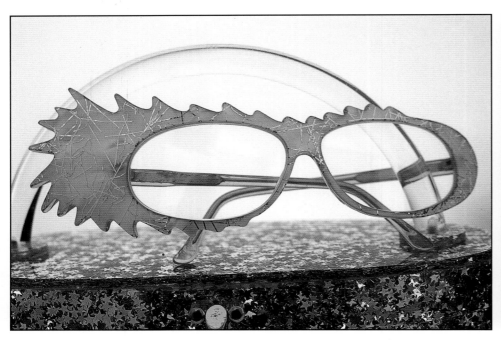

Dreamy iridescent pink and metallic-thread frames, with side sunburst. $300-325.

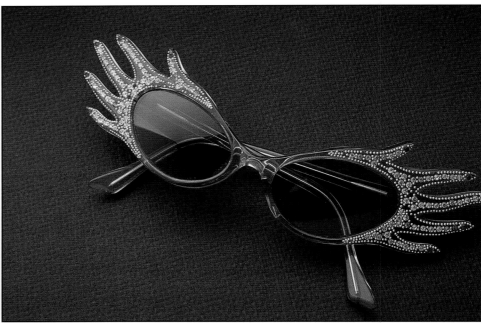

Fanciful fingers: rhinestone "hands" (with jeweled nails) reach from the sides of these black stunners. $400-425.

150

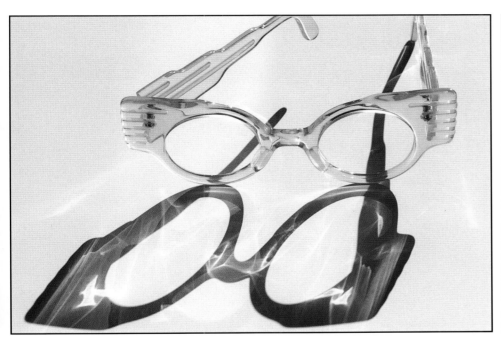

Clearly less menacing: ribbed hinge edges on cool, clear plastic from 1930s Paris. $150-175.

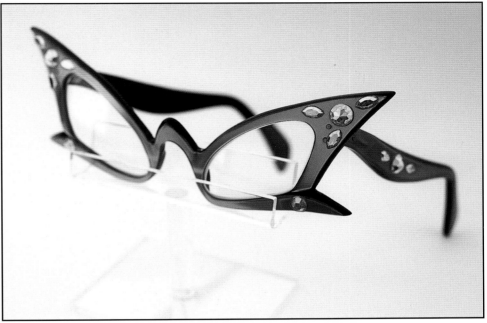

Heading for points unknown: pointy-edge brows in gold, with aurora rhinestones. $325-350.

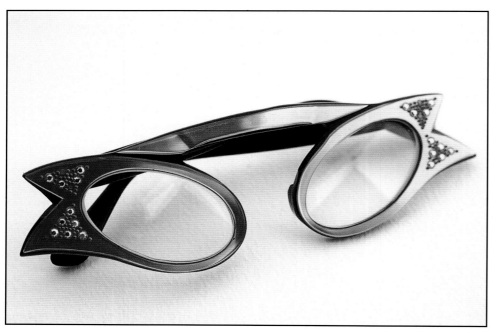

Making more points: double-pointed cat-eyes with aurora rhinestones by Frame France. $200-225.

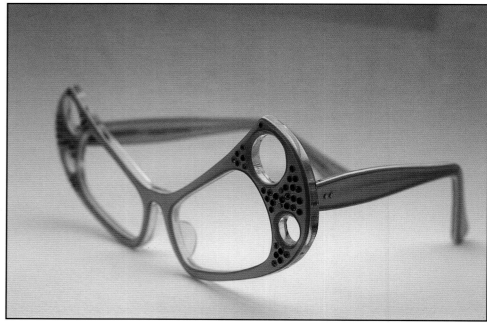

Plush pink, with circular side cutouts. $300-325.

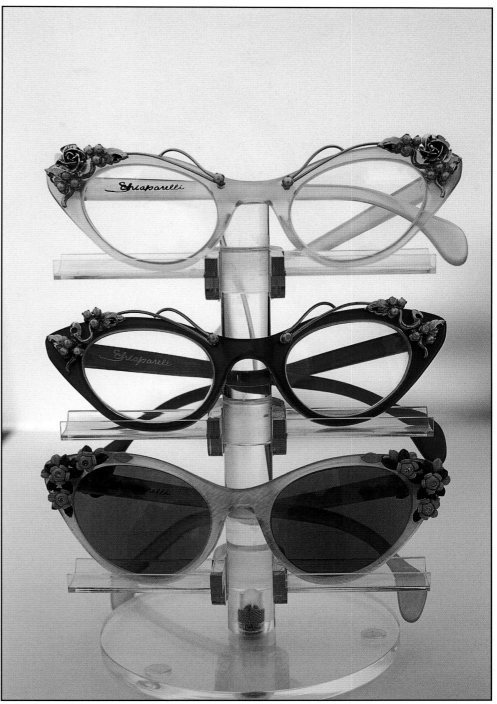

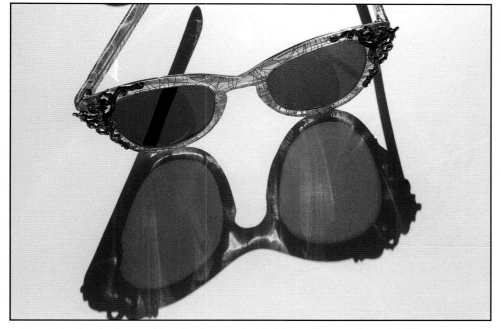

Caught in the shadow: gold and string confetti Schiaparelli wannabes, with filigree embellishments at brow edge. $110-125.

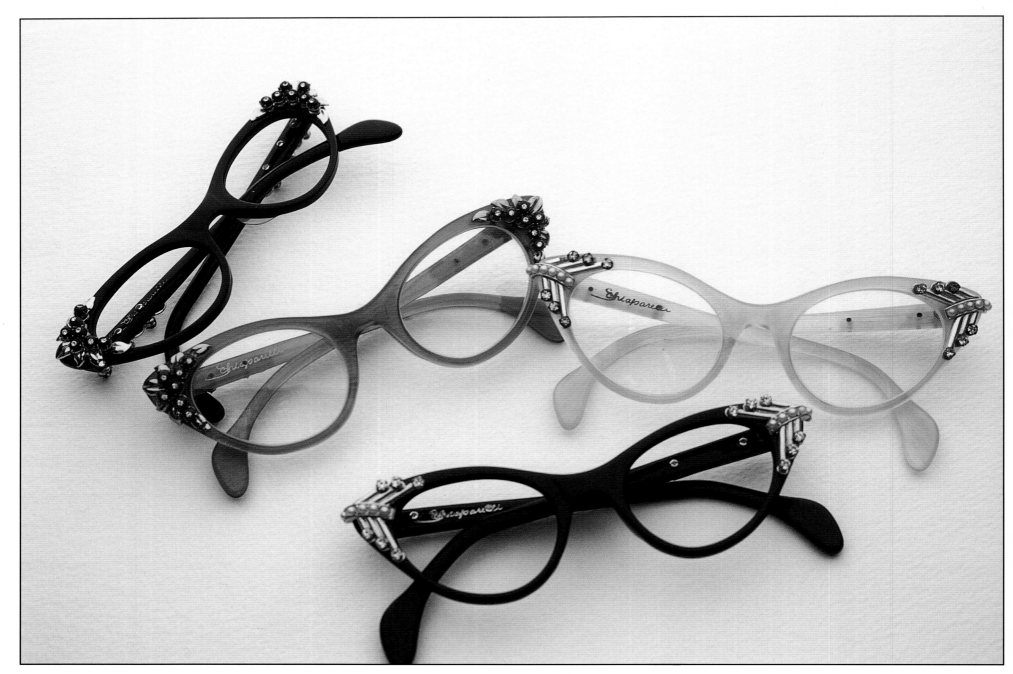

More sumptuous Schiaparellis. $230-250.

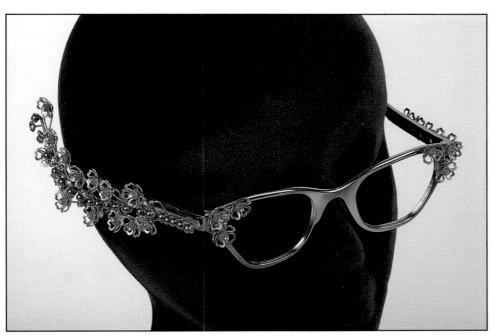

Just right for Roman revels: floral vines at the temple create a wreath-like effect. By Tura, $275-325.

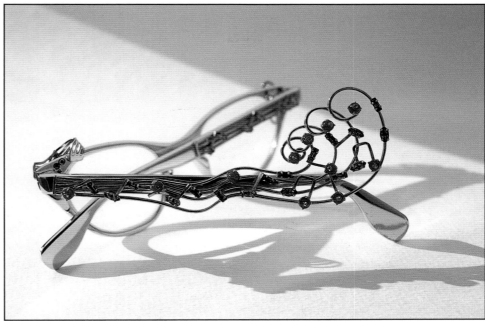

Making a notable impression: also by Tura, these temples feature musical notes and staff. $300-325.

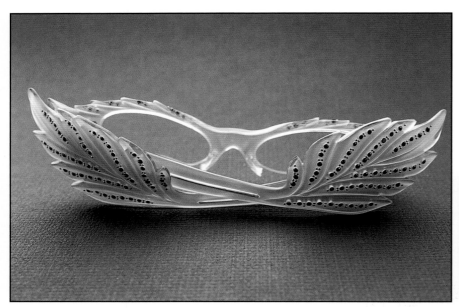

Leaves of jeweled white make attractively inventive earpieces. $400-425.

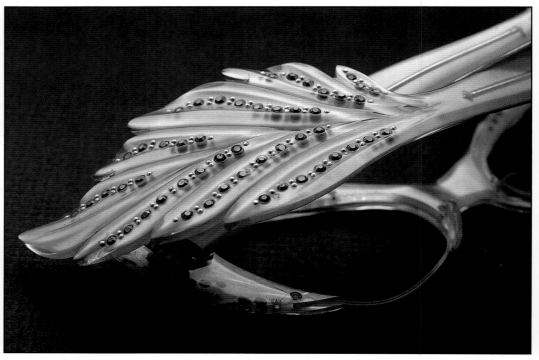

Leaf detail.

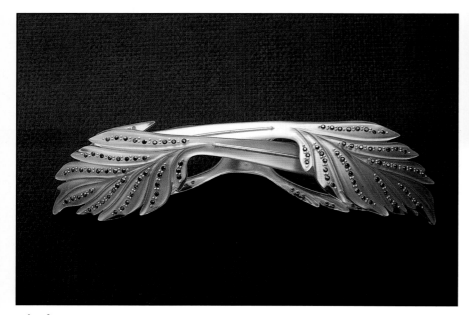

Leafy top view.

Nightwing: gorgeous black butterfly glasses with rhinestone detailing. $350-450.

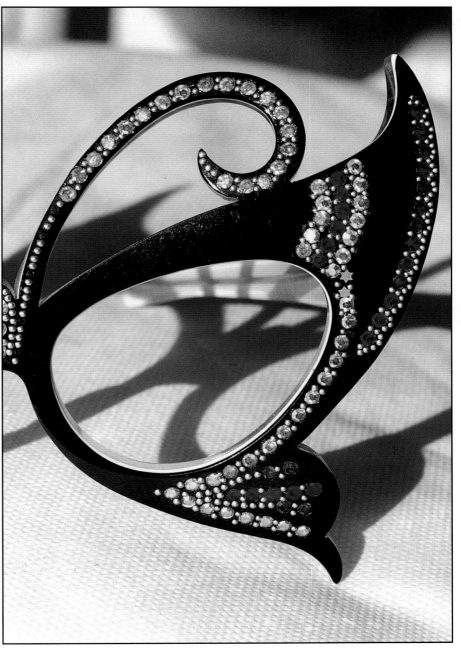

Black butterfly detail.

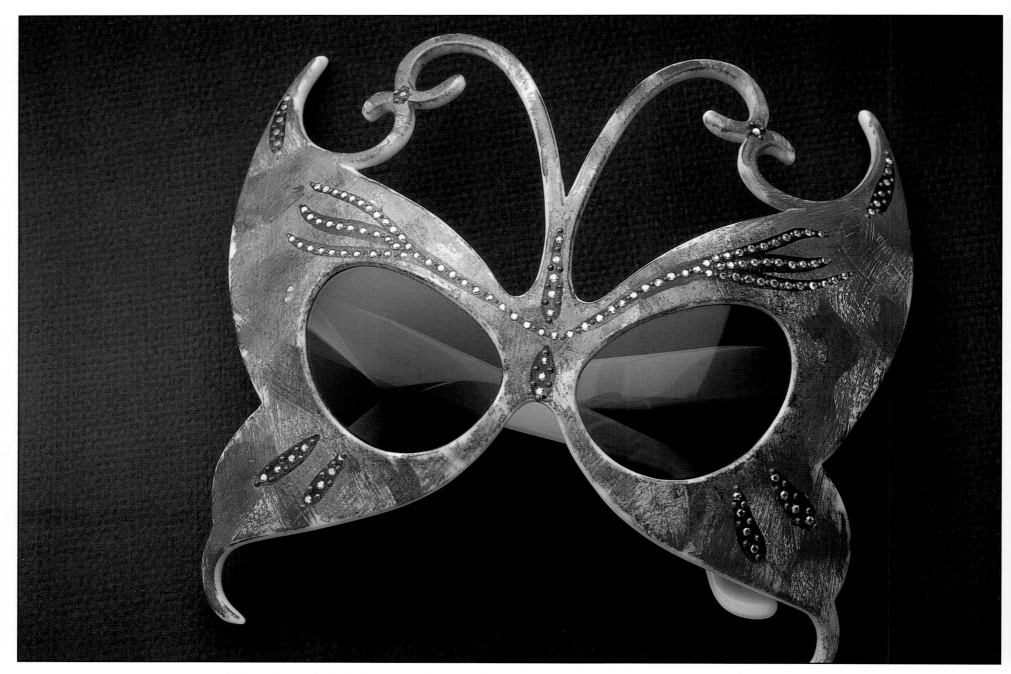

Net results: oversize butterfly glasses with aurora rhinestones, hand painting on cream background. $550-600.

158

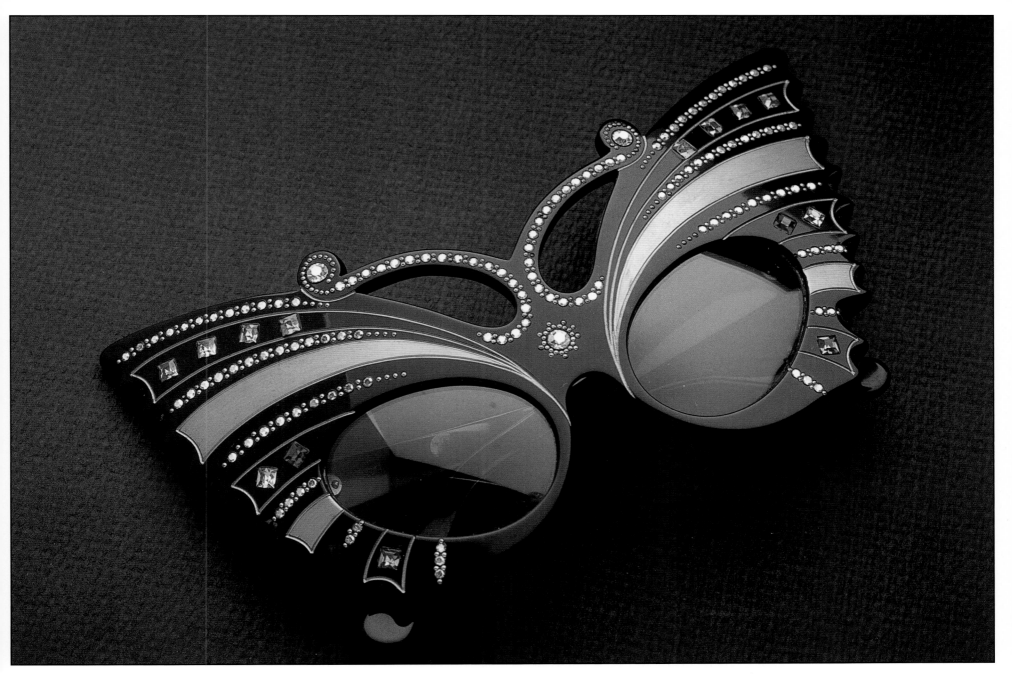

The monarch of all: butterfly glasses with dramatic gold stripes and multi-color square rhinestones on black. $500-550.

Waiting to take flight: ethereal white butterfly glasses with red, blue, and clear rhinestones (plus habitat). $450-475.

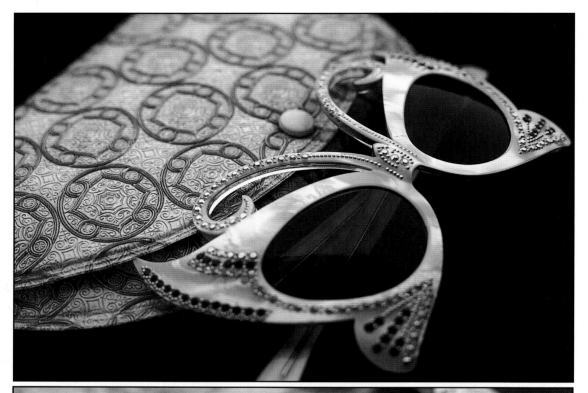

Detail, white butterfly wing.

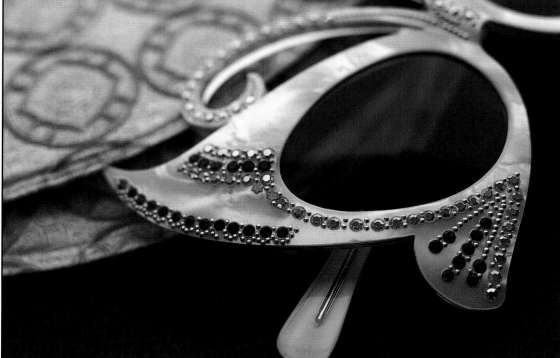

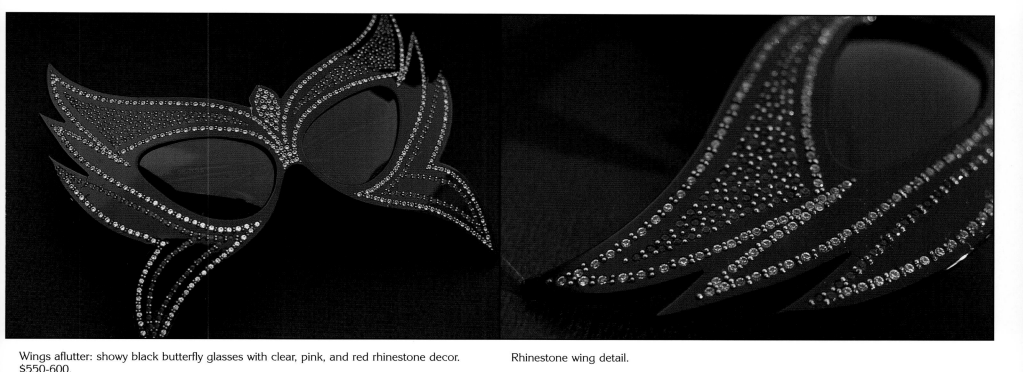

Wings aflutter: showy black butterfly glasses with clear, pink, and red rhinestone decor.
$550-600.

Rhinestone wing detail.

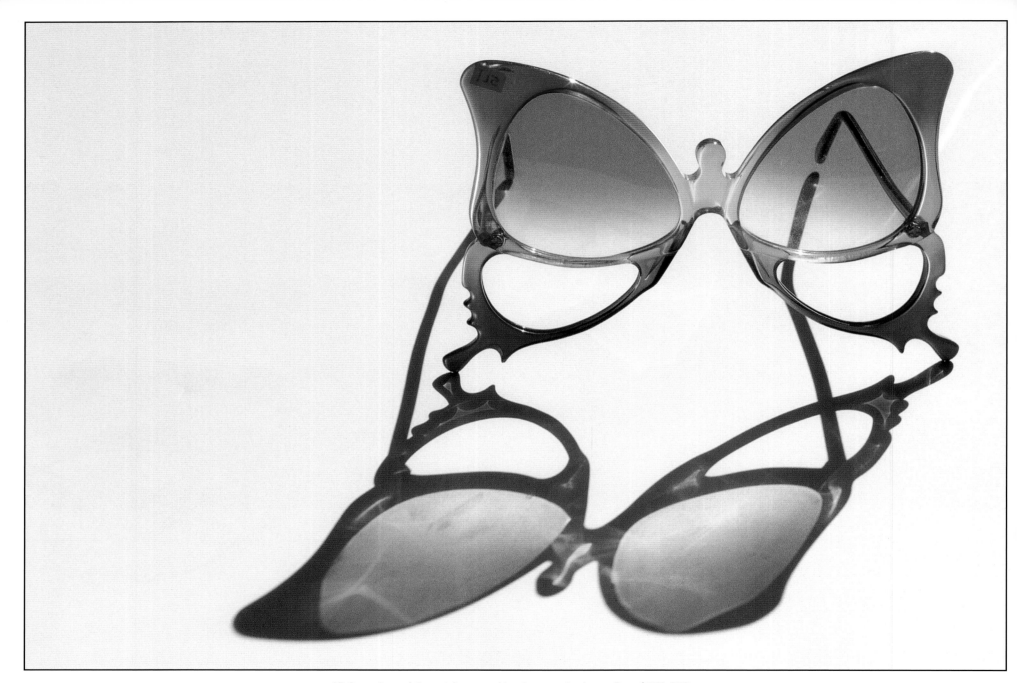

All the colors of the rainbow: multi-color oversize butterflies. $150-250.

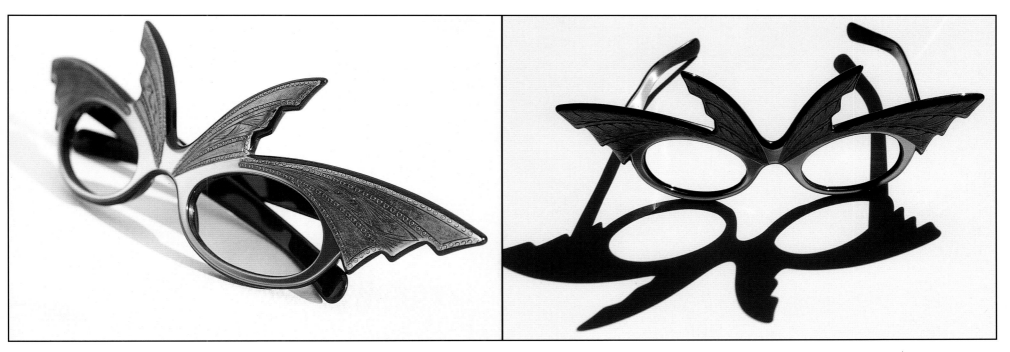

Ideal for Mothra (or Batgirl). "Moth" or "batwing" glasses, in a blend of gentle grays. $375-400.

Break out the mothballs. More moth glasses, with a slightly variant pattern. $375-400.

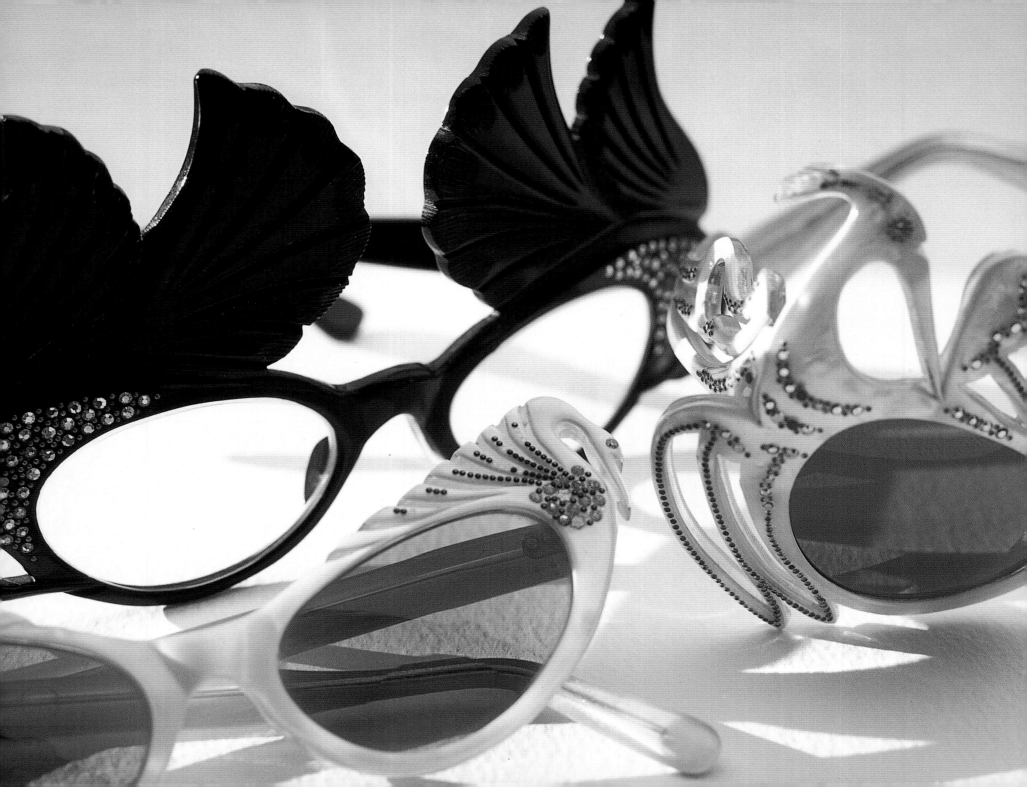

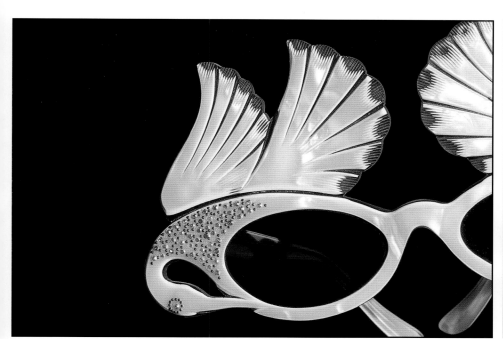 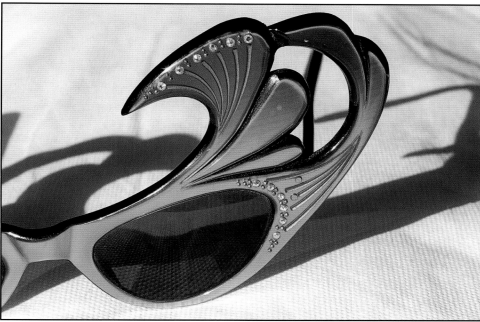

Flight patterns: wing detail of glasses shown on the following pages.

Opposite page:
Taking flight: three soaring "bird wing glasses."
Clockwise from lower left: pearly swans, $200-225;
black swans, $450-550; nesting bird, $600-650.

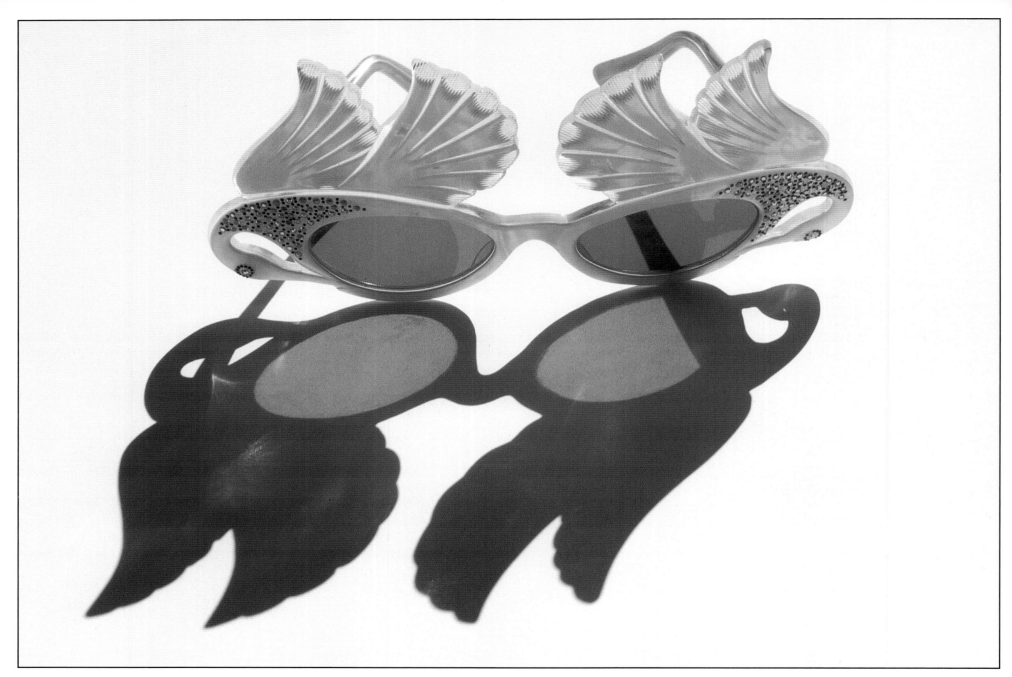

White pearlized swans study their shadows. $450-550.

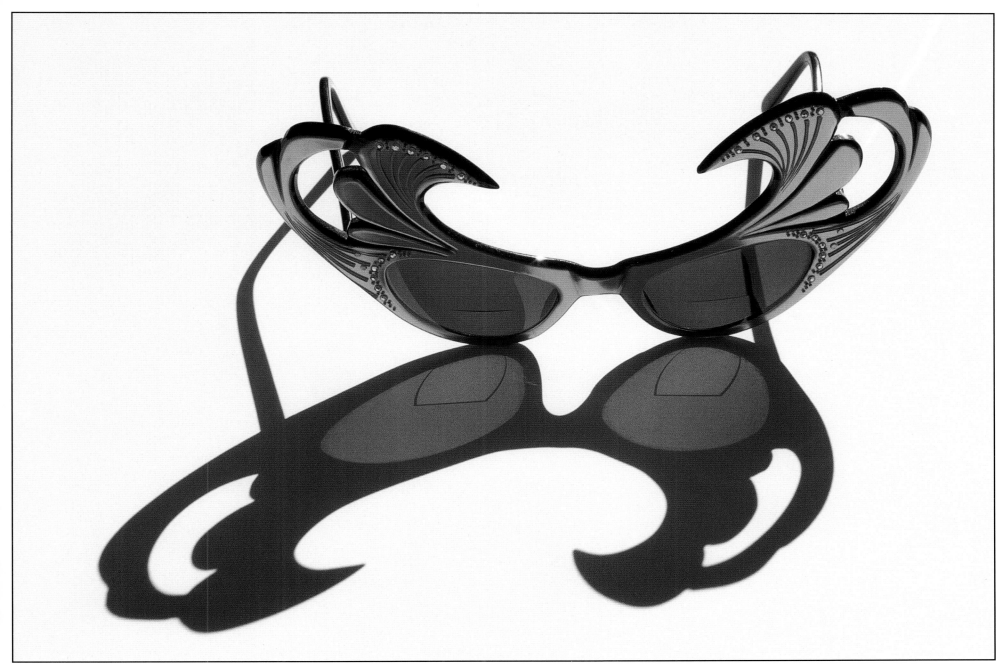

Grand and golden wings. $300-400.

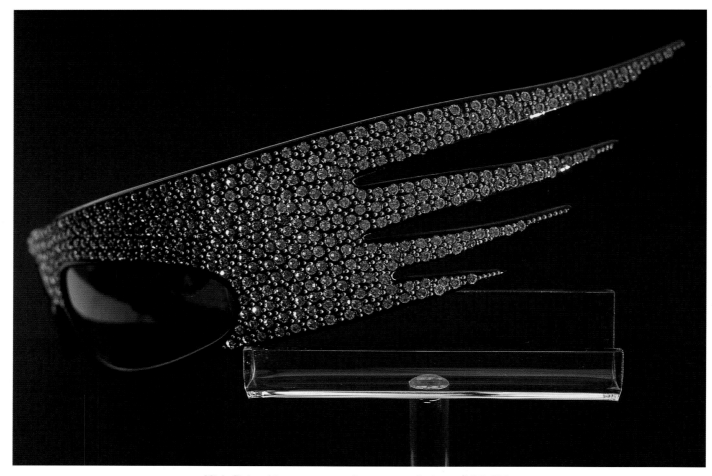

High flight: rhinestone-coated wraparound wings. $550-600.

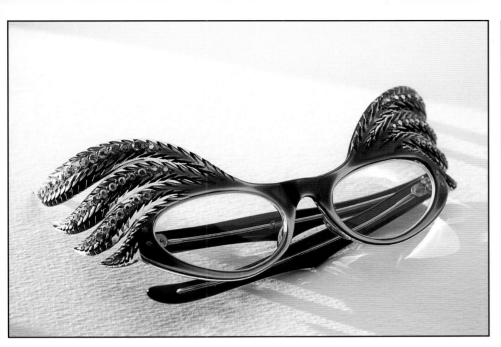

Wings in vivid charcoal and
rhinestone. $450-475.

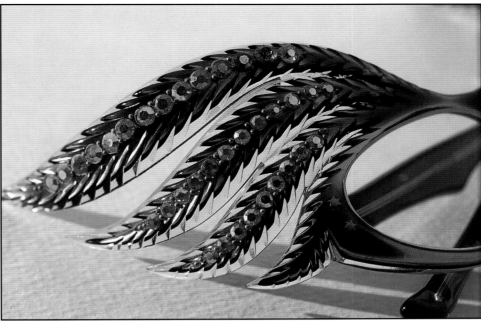

Charcoal and rhinestone detail.

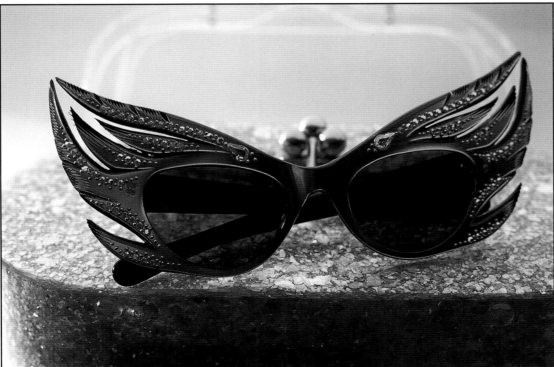

Windswept: black and rhinestone wing arcs. $500-550.

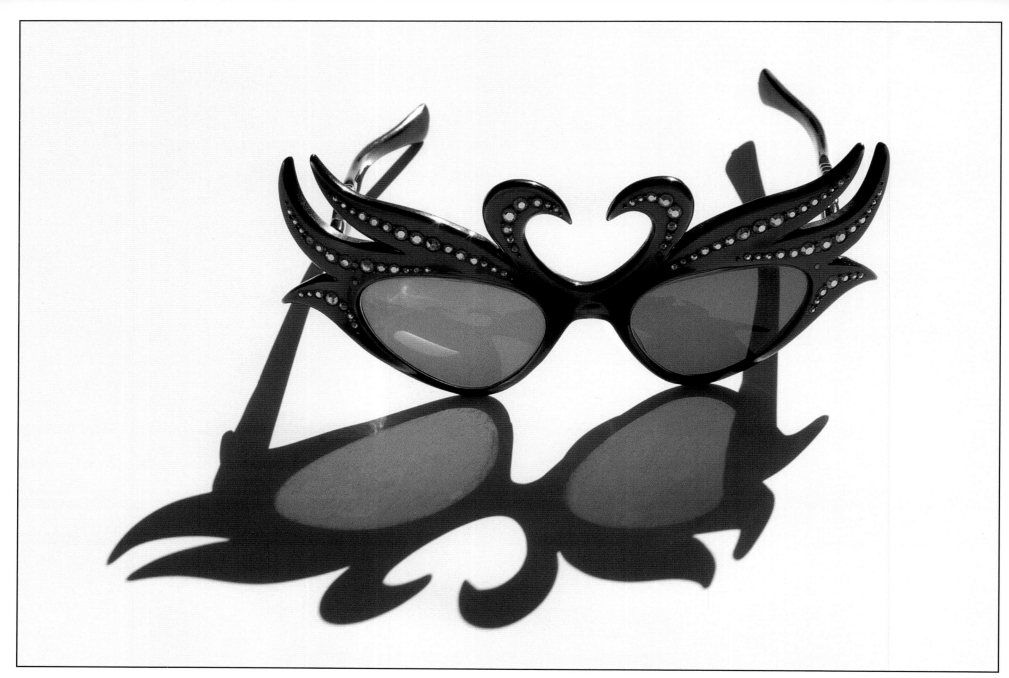

Chocolate-brown wings with rhinestone highlights. $250-350.

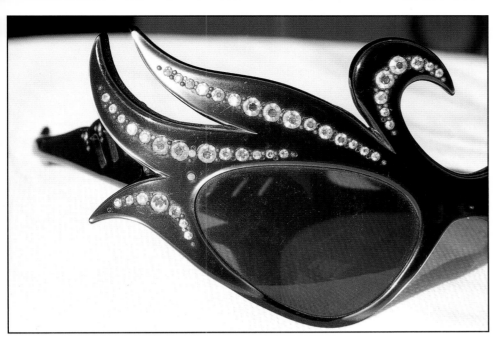

Detail, a study in brown.

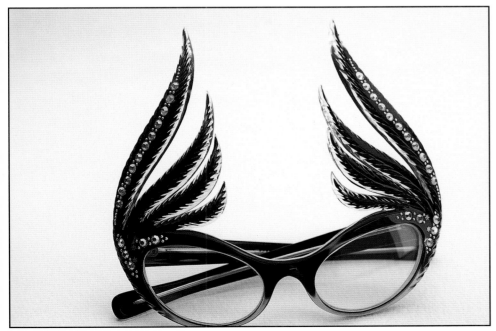

Full sweep: extravagantly arching wings take "specs appeal" to new heights. Black and iridescent gray with aurora rhinestones on outer wing feathers. French, $450-475.

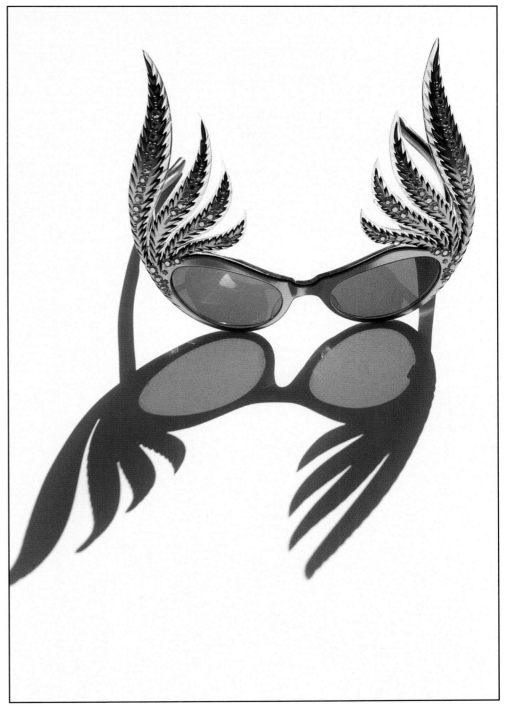

The same, in gray tones with rhinestone embellishment on all feathers. $450-475.

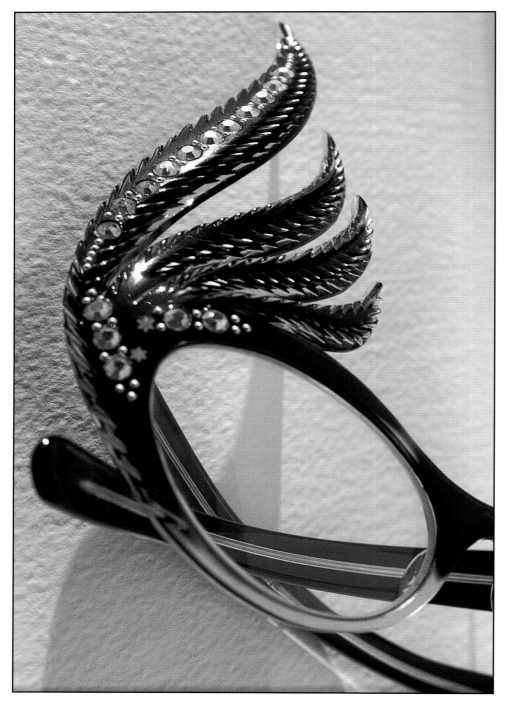

Detail, black high wing.

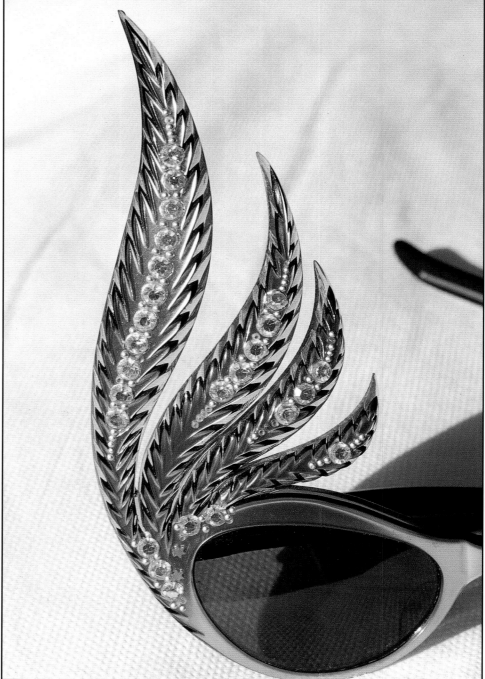

Gray-with-rhinestones high wing detail.

172

Saying good night: "Miss Specs" and her optically enhanced court offer a parting tip of the frames. *Balco News*, July-August, 1955.

See *"On The Cover" Story, Page 31*

Balco News

FOR THE MEN AND WOMEN OF BAUSCH & LOMB OPTICAL COMPANY

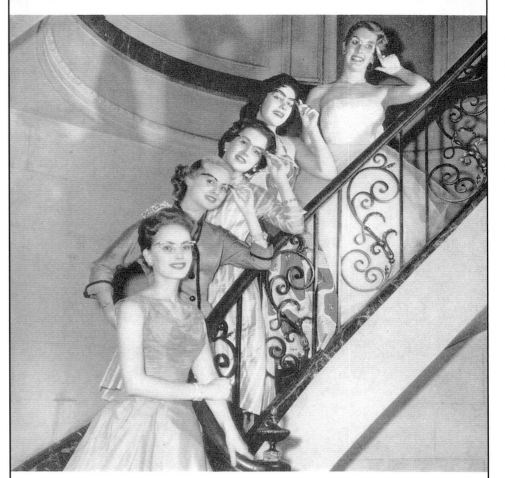

Vol. 15 • No. 4   JULY-AUGUST 1955

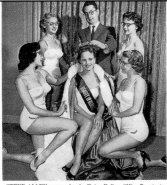

STEVE ALLEN crowns lovely Claire Kallen, "Miss Beauty in Glasses" for 1955 in coronation ceremony at N. Y. press show.

Elect "Miss Beauty in Glasses"

A LOVELY REDHEAD who's worn glasses for 11 years, Claire Kallen of Elizabeth, N. J., is the winner of the third nationwide "Miss Beauty in Glasses" competition.

Crowned queen by TV star Steve Allen at ceremonies in the swank Le Chateau of New York's Savoy Plaza Hotel, she was introduced to millions of people over radio and television as America's most beautiful model who wears glasses.

First in the whirl of activities for vivacious Claire was a day in New York, where she posed for several newsreel and fashion pictures. Immediately after, she spent four days in Rochester, where she

phers Dick Shannon and Kay Conlon, and appeared on a noontime show in the Main dining room.

Following her stay in Rochester, Claire went to Niagara Falls where she modeled the new Ray Ban Caribbean Sun Glasses with the famed waterfalls as a background.

During appearances on the Steve Allen and Dave Garroway television shows in New York, an audience of millions of viewers saw the attractive Conover model demonstrate how different eyewear styles are needed for various activities during the day. Claire, who's also working toward an acting career, modeled the Golden Hi-Lite for

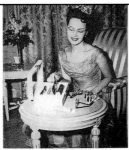

"THEY'RE STUNNING!" exclaims Claire as she views her colorful wardrobe eyeglass frame assortment.

lar Balrim B-31 for business and everyday activity.

On hand for the whirl of activities were Frame Sales Manager Dick Eisenhart and Assistant Advertising manager Ray Van de Vate. Dick crowned "Miss Beauty" at an earlier reception for Warner-Pathé cameramen.

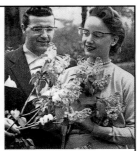

FASHION ESCORT Bob Clark's Keynoter frames and Claire's Hi-Lite styles blend harmoniously with lilacs.

Furthering the purpose of the contest, Claire stated: "The well-dressed woman has a number of frame styles for various occasions and personal needs. They are indispensable to her wardrobe."

The "Miss Beauty in Glasses" Contest was begun to emphasize the "one pair of glasses is not enough" campaign.

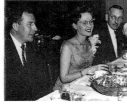

NOONTIME plant dinner finds Claire

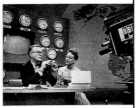

TV STAR Dave Garroway learns im-

Back where we began, with "Miss Beauty in Glasses." Claire Kallen, the winner for 1955, says "the well-dressed woman has a number of frame styles for various occasions and personal needs. They are indispensable to her wardrobe." "Specs Appeal" is here to stay!

BIBLIOGRAPHY

Acerenza, Franca. *Eyewear: Gli Occhiali.* San Francisco, CA: Chronicle Books, 1988.

A New Century. Rochester, NY: Bausch & Lomb, Inc., 1953.

Baron, Julie, ed. *Frames.* Sylmar, CA: Zulch & Zulch, Inc., 1972.

Bronson, Dr. L.D. *Early American Specs.* Glendale, CA: The Occidental Publishing Company, 1974.

"Buddy's Glasses Found." *Rave On!* (April 1980): p. 3.

Butler, Elaine. "Spaghetti Menagerie." *Collectibles: Flea Market Finds* (Spring 1999): pp. 66-70, 77-78.

Chappell, Jennifer. "Sunglasses." *Coastal Living,* no. 4 (July-August 1999): pp. 88-92, 151.

Evans, Mike, ed. *Sunglasses.* New York: Universe Publishing, 1996.

Gaynor, Elizabeth. "Looking Good." *Parade Magazine* (October 17, 1999): pp. 16-19.

Holthaus, Tim, and Jim Petzold, ed. *Ceramic Arts Studio Collectors Price Guide 1997.* Madison, WI: CAS Collectors Association, 1997.

Lahr, John. *Dame Edna Everage and the Rise of Western Civilization.* New York: Farrar Straus Giroux, 1992.

Mattison-Shupnick, Matt, and others. *Hindsight: Sola Celebrates the History of Eyewear.* Sunnyvale, CA: Sola Optical USA, 1995.

McKinnon, Lisa. "Vintage Eyewear." *The Star, Ventura* (September 26, 1997): pp. C1, C8.

Nicola, Gloria, ed. "Flashback: Then and Now." *20/20* September, 1997: pp. 56-63.

Patteson, Jean. "Barbie Eyeglasses For Big Girls." *The Orlando Sentinel* (March 30, 1999)

Perec, Georges and Yves Hersant, photography by Timothy Street Porter. "Hollywood On Eyes." *FMR America 3* (August 1984): pp. 95-105.

Rosenkrantz, Linda. "Contemporary Collectibles: Eyewear Collection Can Be Quite A Spectacle." *Antique Journal* (June 2000): pp. 21-22.

Rosenthal, J. William, M.D. *Spectacles and Other Vision Aids: A History and Guide to Collecting.* San Francisco: Norman Publishing, 1996.

St. Michael, Mick. *Elton John.* New York: Smithmark Publisher Inc., 1994.

Schiffer, Nancy N. *Eyeglass Retrospective: Where Fashion Meets Science.* Atglen, PA: Schiffer Publishing, 2000.

"The Evolution Of An Industry: Glimpses Into Days Gone By." *Eyecare Business* (December, 1999): pp. 19-20.

United States Patent Office *Official Gazette,* 1945-1975.

Whitman, Anne. "Retro-Specs." *Eyecare Business* (December 1999): pp. 41-59.

Periodicals and Catalogs (advertisements and product announcements)

American Optical Company catalogs; Balco News; Business Week; McCall's; The Optical Journal; The Optometric Weekly; The Saturday Evening Post; Selecta Frames catalogs; Spencer Optical Manufacturing Co. catalogs; Seventeen; The Western Optical World; Vogue; Woman's Home Companion

INDEX

Additional Photo Credits

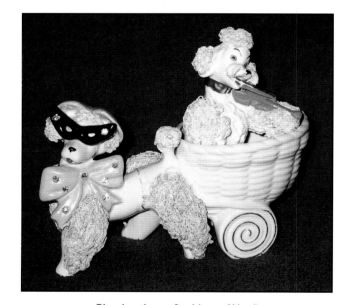

Glenda takes a final bow. (Wow!)

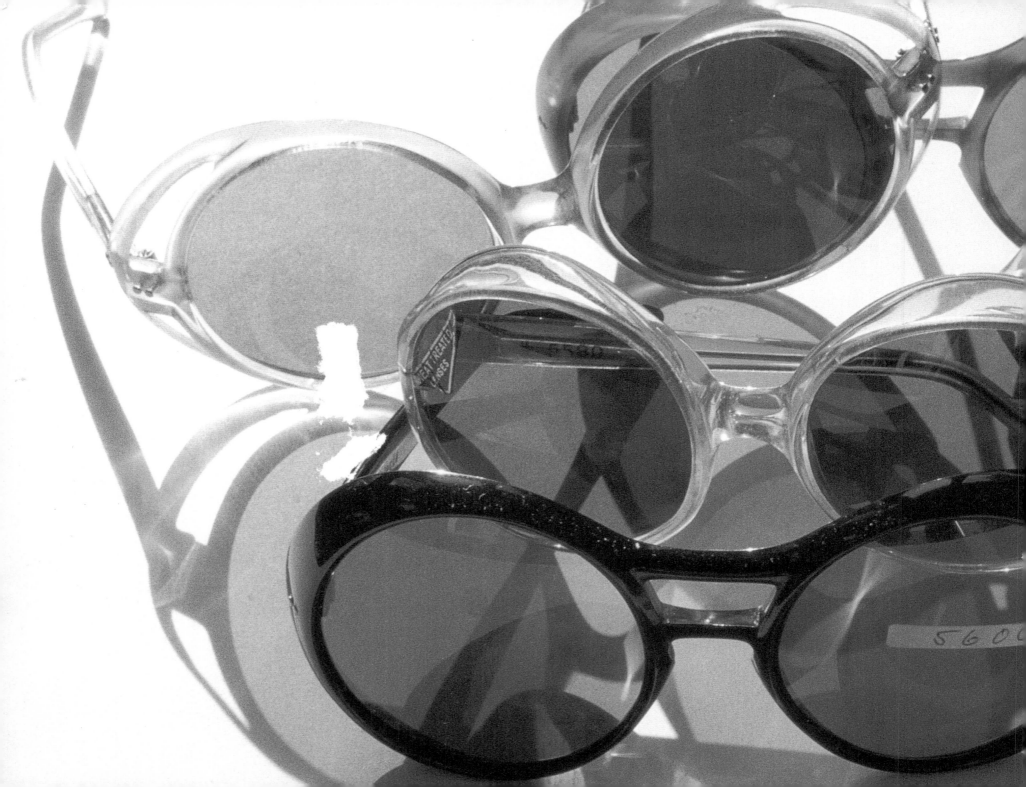